HOW TO TRANSFORM YOUR LIFE WITH CHAIR YOGA

Say goodbye to aches and pains with chair yoga

TONY D. SPAULDING

Table of Contents

INTRODUCTION

CHAPTER 1
What is it about Chair Yoga
Seniors' Chair Yoga Exercise
Ten Benefits of Chair Yoga and How to Do It
Chair Yoga Equipment Required

CHAPER 2
Essential Stretching Exercises for Seniors to
Do Every Day
9 Essential Stretching Exercises for Seniors
to Do Every Day
Genie Stretching

CHAPTER 3
Basic and Core Strength Exercises
Basic Strength Exercises for Men
Exercises that will improve your health
Weekly schedule of chair yoga exercises

CHAPTER 4
Strength Training Exercise for Elderly in 20 Minutes
Chair Yoga Training Plan
A Beginner's Guide to Strengthening
The Elements of a Successful Workout

CHAPTER 5
How Chair Yoga can Help You

CHAPTER 6
Workout for Well-Being.
Physical Benefits of Working Out
Mental Benefits of Working Out
General pain and recovery core workout for seniors
Exercises to Perform If You Have Back Pain
How to improve the strength of your core and glutes.
Weight Loss Workout Guide
Workout for Knee Injury
Wheel chair workout

CHAPTER 7
Physical, Mental and Emotional Benefits of Chair Yoga
Emotional Benefits of Chair Yoga

Conclusion

INTRODUCTION

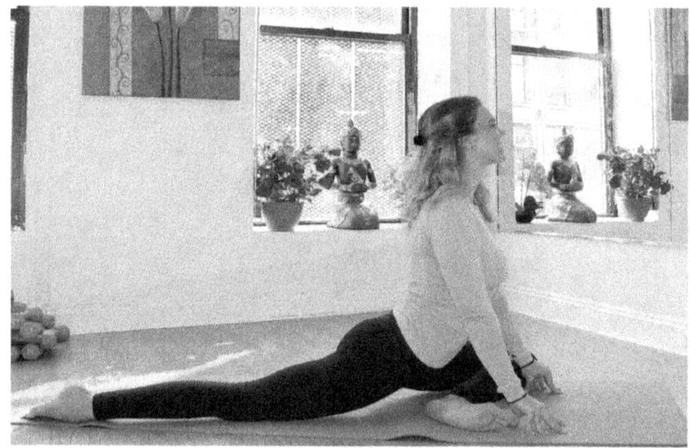

Chair yoga is a form of yoga that is designed specifically for seniors or individuals with limited mobility. It is a low-impact form of exercise that can be done while seated in a chair or while using the chair for support. The benefits of chair yoga for seniors are numerous, including increased flexibility, improved balance, reduced stress, and improved overall health and well-being.

One of the biggest benefits of chair yoga is that it is a low-impact form of exercise. This means that seniors can participate in chair yoga without putting unnecessary strain on their joints and muscles. This is particularly important for seniors who may have health conditions such as arthritis, joint pain, or weak bones.

In addition to being low-impact, chair yoga is also highly accessible. Unlike traditional yoga, which requires a certain level of physical ability and mobility, chair yoga can be done by anyone, regardless of their fitness level or physical abilities. This makes it an ideal form of exercise for seniors who may have difficulty getting up and down from the floor or who have limited mobility in their arms or legs.

One of the key benefits of chair yoga is that it can help improve flexibility and balance. As we age, our muscles and joints naturally become stiffer, making it more difficult to move around and perform everyday tasks. Chair yoga helps to counter this by providing a gentle and effective way to increase flexibility and improve balance. This is especially important for seniors, who are at an increased risk of falls and other types of accidents due to their decreased mobility.

Another benefit of chair yoga is that it can help reduce stress and improve mental well-being. Yoga has been shown to have a positive effect on mental health, helping to reduce anxiety and depression and improve overall mood. This is especially important for seniors, who may be dealing with the physical and emotional challenges that come with aging.

Finally, chair yoga can also help improve overall health and well-being. By promoting flexibility, balance, and reducing stress, chair yoga can help seniors maintain a healthy and active lifestyle, reducing their risk of health problems and promoting overall physical and mental wellness.

Chair yoga is a safe and effective form of exercise for seniors. It offers numerous benefits, including increased flexibility, improved balance, reduced stress, and improved overall health and well-being. Whether you are a senior who is new to yoga or an experienced yogi looking to modify your practice, chair yoga is a great way to stay active, healthy, and happy as you age.

CHAPTER 1

What is it about Chair Yoga

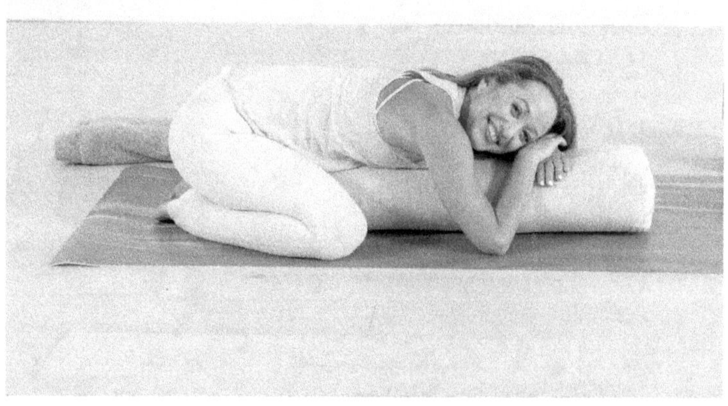

Yoga is a practice that has been around for thousands of years, and it has been adapted in many ways to accommodate various populations and conditions. Chair yoga is one such adaptation that has gained popularity in recent years. It is a modified form of traditional yoga that is performed while sitting on a chair. In this book, we will explore the specific conditions and populations that can benefit from chair yoga.

For Older Adults

Chair yoga is an ideal form of exercise for older adults. As we age, our bodies become less flexible and more prone to injury, making traditional yoga poses difficult to perform. Chair yoga offers many of the same benefits as traditional yoga, such as improved flexibility, strength, and balance, but with modifications that make it safe and accessible for older adults. Chair yoga can also help to reduce the risk of falls, which is a major concern for older adults.

For Individuals with Limited Mobility

Chair yoga is also an excellent option for individuals with limited mobility. Whether due to injury, disability, or chronic pain, traditional yoga poses may be too difficult or even impossible to perform. Chair yoga offers a way to practice yoga in a seated position, with modifications that can be tailored to individual needs. This makes it possible for individuals with limited mobility to experience the benefits of yoga, such as improved flexibility and strength.

For Individuals with Chronic Pain

Chair yoga can also be beneficial for individuals with chronic pain. Many traditional yoga poses can put a strain on the joints, which can exacerbate pain. Chair yoga, on the other hand, is gentler and less demanding on the body. It can help to reduce pain by improving flexibility and strength, as well as promoting relaxation and stress reduction.

For Individuals with Mental Health Conditions

Chair yoga can also be helpful for individuals with mental health conditions, such as anxiety and depression. Yoga has been shown to have a positive impact on mental health by reducing stress and promoting relaxation. Chair yoga can be especially helpful because it is accessible and can be done in a variety of settings, making it a convenient way to incorporate yoga into a mental health treatment plan.

Chair yoga is a modified form of traditional yoga that can provide many benefits to a variety of populations and conditions. Whether you are an older adult, have limited mobility, chronic pain, or a mental health condition, chair yoga offers a safe and accessible way to practice yoga and improve your overall health and well-being.

Seniors' Chair Yoga Exercise

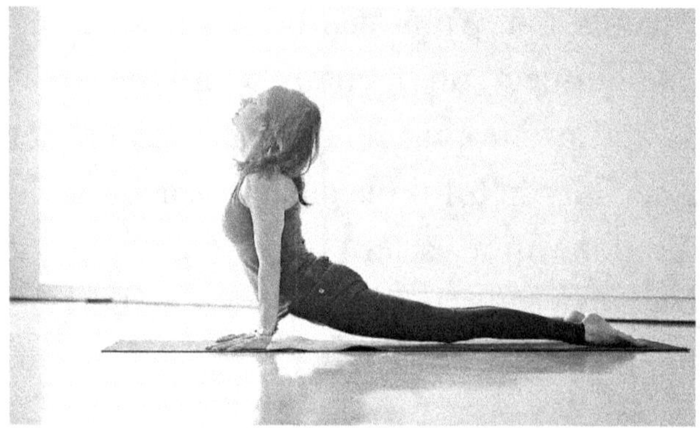

Chair yoga is specifically designed for seniors or individuals with limited mobility. By using a chair as support, this form of yoga provides seniors with a safe and effective way to improve flexibility, balance, and overall health. In this article, we will explore the numerous benefits of chair yoga for seniors and why it is an ideal form of exercise for this population.

First and foremost, chair yoga is a low-impact form of exercise, making it an ideal choice for seniors who may have health conditions such as arthritis, joint pain, or weak bones. Unlike traditional yoga, which requires a certain level of physical ability and mobility, chair yoga can be performed by anyone, regardless of their fitness level or physical abilities. This is particularly beneficial for seniors who may have difficulty getting up and down from the floor or who have limited mobility in their arms or legs.

One of the key benefits of chair yoga is that it can help improve flexibility and balance. As we age, our muscles and joints naturally become stiffer, making it more difficult to move around and perform everyday tasks. Chair yoga provides a gentle and effective way to increase flexibility and improve balance, reducing the risk of falls and other types of accidents.

In addition to improving physical health, chair yoga can also have a positive impact on mental well-being. Yoga has been shown to have a calming effect on the mind and body, reducing stress, anxiety, and depression. For seniors, this can be particularly beneficial as they may be dealing with the physical and emotional challenges that come with aging.

Furthermore, chair yoga is a highly accessible form of exercise. All you need is a chair, making it easy to participate in yoga from the comfort of your own home. This is especially important for seniors who may have difficulty getting to and from a gym or yoga studio.

Chair yoga is a safe and effective form of exercise for seniors. Whether you are a senior who is new to yoga or an experienced yogi looking to modify your practice, chair yoga is a great way to stay active, healthy, and happy as you age. With its numerous benefits, including improved flexibility, balance, and mental well-being, chair yoga is an ideal form of exercise for seniors and is well worth considering as a part of a healthy and active lifestyle.

Chair yoga is a gentle form of yoga that is perfect for seniors who want to stay active and improve their flexibility, strength, and balance. This type of yoga is performed while seated in a chair, making it accessible for those who have limited mobility or are unable to stand for long periods of time.

One of the benefits of chair yoga is that it provides a low-impact workout that is easy on the joints. This makes it an excellent option for seniors who may be dealing with conditions such as arthritis, osteoporosis, or other joint pain. The slow, controlled movements of chair yoga also help to reduce the risk of falls and increase balance.

In addition to the physical benefits, chair yoga can also help seniors to reduce stress and improve their overall sense of well-being. The deep breathing and mindfulness practices that are a part of yoga can help to calm the mind and improve mental clarity, which can be especially beneficial for seniors who may be dealing with anxiety or depression.

Here are some of the most common chair yoga exercises for seniors:

Seated Cat-Cow: Start by sitting in a chair with your feet flat on the floor and your hands resting on your knees. Inhale and lift your chin and chest towards the ceiling, then exhale and round your spine, bringing your chin to your chest. Repeat this movement several times, moving slowly and smoothly.

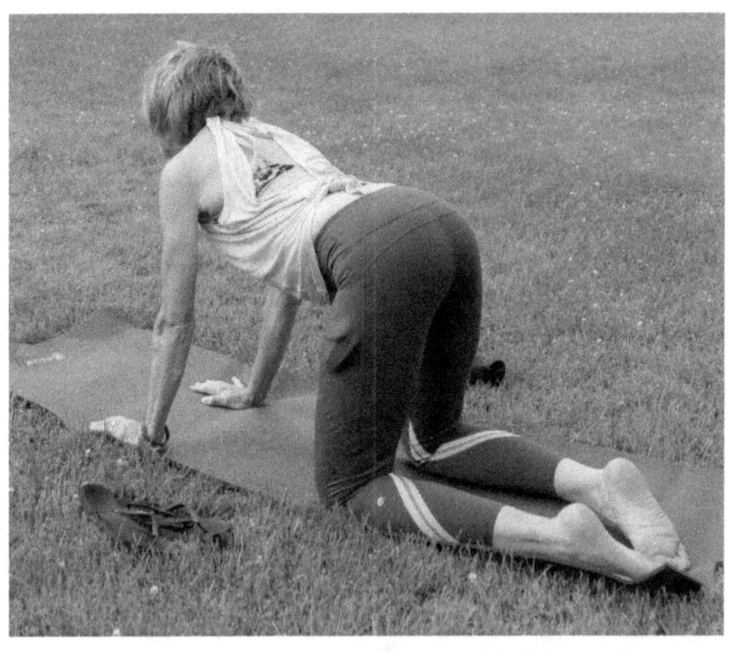

Seated Twist: Start by sitting in a chair with your feet flat on the floor. Place your left hand on your right knee and your right hand on the back of the chair. Inhale and twist your torso to the right, then exhale and release. Repeat on the other side.

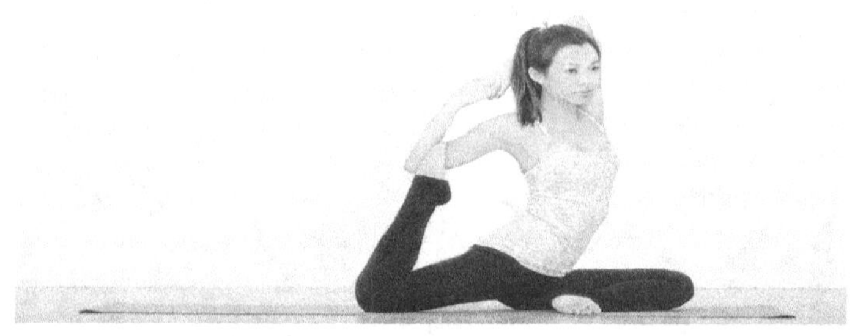

Seated Mountain: Start by sitting in a chair with your feet flat on the floor. Place your hands on your knees and sit up straight, imagining that there is a string attached to the top of your head that is pulling you up toward the ceiling. Hold this position for several deep breaths, then release.

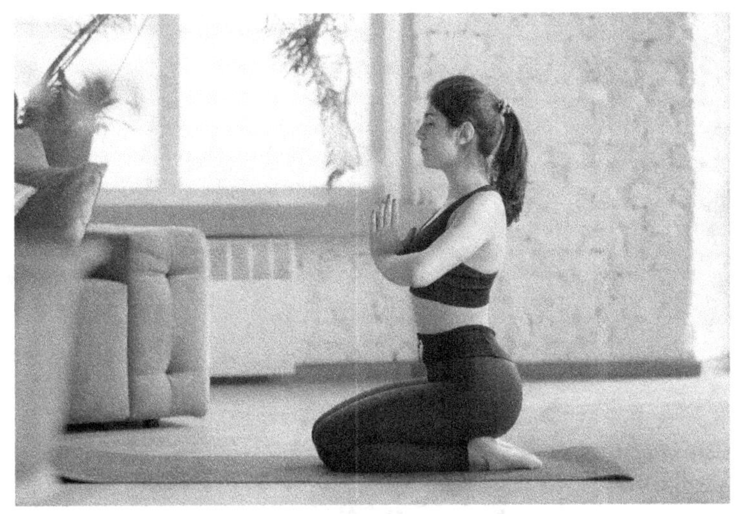

Seated Shoulder Shrugs: Start by sitting in a chair with your feet flat on the floor. Inhale and lift your shoulders towards your ears, then exhale and release. Repeat several times, moving slowly and smoothly.

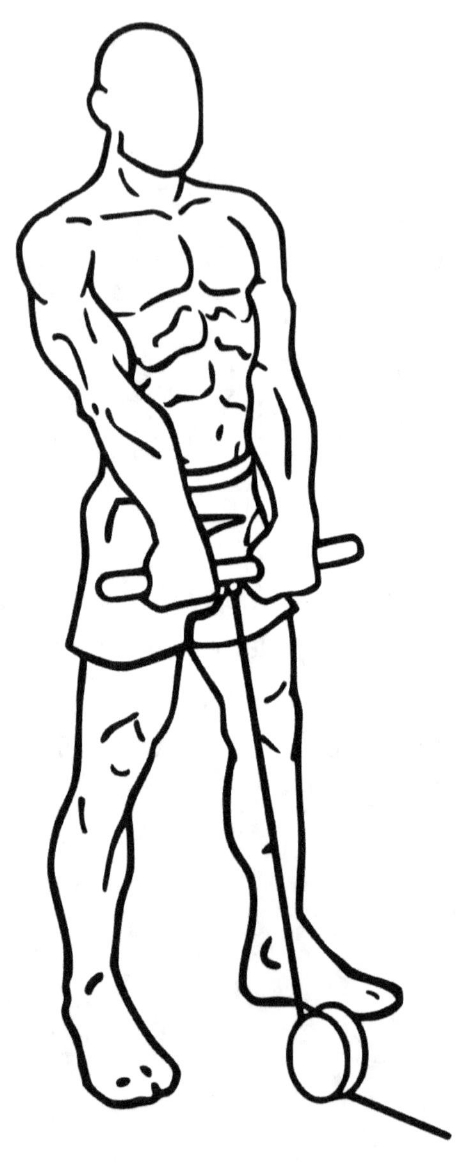

Seated Arm Stretches: Start by sitting in a chair with your feet flat on the floor. Reach one arm up towards the ceiling, then lean over to the side and stretch the arm across your body. Repeat on the other side.

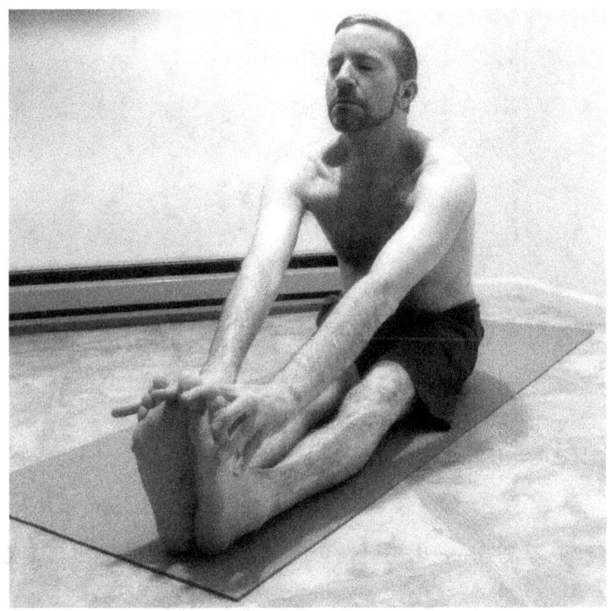

__Seated Leg Lifts__: Start by sitting in a chair with your feet flat on the floor. Inhale and lift one leg off the ground, then exhale and release. Repeat several times on each leg.

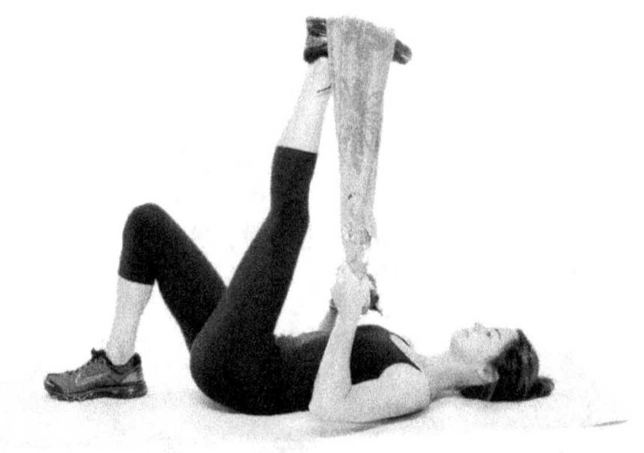

It's important to note that before starting any new exercise regimen, it's always a good idea to consult with your doctor to make sure that it's safe for you. If you experience any pain or discomfort during these exercises, stop and consult with your doctor.

Chair yoga is a great way for seniors to stay active, improve their physical and mental well-being, and reduce the risk of falls and other injuries. With its gentle, low-impact movements, chair yoga is an accessible and effective form of exercise for seniors of all abilities.

Ten Benefits of Chair Yoga and How to Do It

A chair yoga sequence may surprise you, but it is one of the most useful types of yoga sequences to have at your disposal. What are the benefits of doing chair yoga, and how can you get started?

This book will teach you about the ten advantages of practicing chair yoga. As well as advice and tips on how to best practice.

Benefits of Chair Yoga

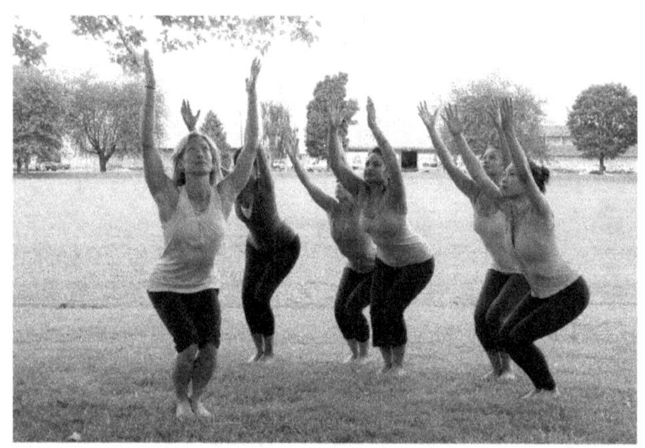

Why Should You Do It?

1. Chair yoga is for everyone, regardless of age or physical ability.

The majority of people can do gentle chair yoga sequences. "If you can breathe, you can do yoga," says T. Krishnamacharya (often referred to as the great-grandfather of yoga).

Recently, photos of beautiful young models and dancers in advanced, pretzel-like yoga poses have gained popularity on social media. Unfortunately, this can give newcomers to yoga the impression that they must be fit, flexible, and strong. Yoga is, in fact, a practice that can be tailored to each individual's needs.

Your physical health, fitness level, wealth, or location have no bearing on your ability to practice yoga. It is also not necessary to have an expensive yoga mat, fashionable clothing, or access to a yoga studio.

Chair yoga is beneficial to everyone. From those of us who work in an office or at home behind a computer to those of us who are injured or elderly. If you work regularly behind a desk, chair yoga exercises can be easily incorporated into your workday. You only need a 5 - 15 minute break from work to practice a short chair yoga sequence.

If you have an injury, have limited mobility, or are a senior, chair yoga poses will be much more accessible than standing and lying yoga poses in a Hatha, Vinyasa, or Ashtanga yoga practice.

You will be able to use the chair as a prop and modify yoga poses to fit your body better. Yoga in a chair allows you to work in a safe way to open and strengthen your body while also relaxing your mind.

2. Improve your overall health by incorporating more movement into your daily routine.

The majority of us lead sedentary lives, spending the majority of our time sitting. This can include reading, using a computer, traveling, and watching TV during our work hours. There is mounting evidence that, unless you are in a wheelchair, excessive sitting can be harmful to your health.

We can improve our overall health by being more physically active and adding more movement to our days. It's no surprise, then, that the UK National Health Service (NHS) recommends that we engage in some form of physical activity every day.

Physical activity of any kind is beneficial, and the more you do, the better. If you can find a type of movement that you enjoy, you will be more likely to engage in it and thus be in better overall health.

To reduce our risk of illness from inactivity, we should exercise regularly, at least 150 minutes per week, and limit our sitting time.

The UK Chief Medical Officers' Physical Activity Guidelines report suggests breaking up long periods of sitting with one to two minutes of activity. Being physically active every day lays the groundwork for a healthier and happier life.

Chair yoga allows you to incorporate more gentle and low-impact movements into your day. Short chair yoga sequences can be used to break up long periods of sitting throughout the day.

People frequently believe that they must set aside significant amounts of time to engage in physical activity. Chair yoga requires only a few minutes of practice. Making it easier to incorporate more movement into your day.

3. Release tension in your body caused by long periods of sitting. So we've concluded that the majority of us spend a lot of time sitting and that adding some gentle movement into our day with chair yoga can be very beneficial.

You've probably noticed physical tension building up in your body after sitting for long periods of time. Slumping in our seats, face muscles contracted, neck leaning forward, shoulders high, and back rounded, we can begin to lose our good posture.

It's not surprising that minor aches and pains can escalate into long-term tension and pain. This causes headaches, chronic neck and shoulder pain, and excruciating back pain.

You can relieve some of the tension and tightness that has built up from sitting for long periods of time by taking a short break in your day to do chair yoga.

Chair yoga allows you to specifically target areas of tightness in your face, neck, shoulders, and back. And discover that by bringing more mobility and strength to these areas, you can aid your pains and reduce tension in your body as you practice regularly.

4. Improve your physical well-being, sleep better, and reduce pain.

Our physical well-being is critical for making the most of our lives. It includes not only being disease-free but also having enough energy throughout the day. Can we accomplish everything we want during the day without becoming exhausted or physically depleted?

The UK National Health Service (NHS) mentions evidence that a regular yoga practice is beneficial for people with high blood pressure, heart disease, aches and pains, including lower back, shoulder, and neck pain.

Physical Activity Guidelines report suggests that light forms of exercise, such as chair yoga, can help improve the quality of our sleep and help us maintain a healthy weight.

These advantages of feeling better rested, less in pain, and less susceptible to illness will make it easier to be more active and enjoy life.

As a result, chair yoga has the potential to give us more energy and allow us to do more of the things we want to do during the day.

5. Improve your flexibility and range of motion.

As we age, our bodies become less flexible. If we sit for long periods of time and/or do repetitive activities like walking, cycling, and running, we can develop stiffness and a limited range of mobility earlier in life.

Stretching is therefore an important aspect of yoga to ensure that we have a wide range of mobility as we get older. Allowing us to move freely and remain independent as we age.

Yoga is a safe and effective way to increase flexibility, strength, and balance.

Chair yoga incorporates gentle movements that stretch the body. This helps the body become more flexible, which can help offset the loss of flexibility that occurs as we age.

It takes time and consistency to develop flexibility. So, to improve your range of motion, try doing a little chair yoga on a regular basis.

6. Increase your muscle mass and bone density to become stronger.

Physical strength in our muscles and bones is essential at all ages. From the need to build muscle and bone density earlier in life to maintaining strength throughout adulthood, to postponing the natural decline in muscle strength and bone density as we get older.

To ensure we are literally strong enough to face life, the Physical Activity Guidelines of the Health Council of the Netherlands recommend that all adults work on building strength at least two days a week to keep muscles, bones, and joints strong.

Chair yoga exercises that use your own body weight can help you build or maintain muscle and bone strength.

Chair yoga teaches you how to engage and activate your muscles while also creating additional length and space through stretching.

Chair yoga allows you to use a wide range of muscles in your body, many of which are not used on a regular basis in other activities.

7. Improve your balance and decrease your chances of falling.

Increased balance, as well as flexibility and strength, is beneficial at all stages of life. It can help us move more safely in unpredictable situations and prevent accidents. This is especially important in later life, when improved balance can reduce the risk of frailty and falls.

The Physical Activity Guidelines of the Health Council of the Netherlands recommend that you work on your balance at least twice a week using tools such as yoga.

Balancing in a chair yoga pose is, of course, easier than some of the more traditional standing yoga poses, such as standing on one leg for Vrksasana (the tree pose). However, there are still ways to test your balance while doing chair yoga.

Experiment with changing your center of balance and gravity. While sitting in your chair, experiment with leaning forward, back, or to the side.

Did you feel like different parts of your body had to work together to keep you balanced? Maybe in your feet, legs, and belly?

You've probably noticed that even if you stay seated, the rest of your body has to adapt with balance to keep you steady on the chair.

By repeating these movements on a regular basis, you can help train your body to react to unexpected movements and improve your balance.

8. Relieve stress and provide peace of mind

Chair yoga can benefit your mental health as well as your physical health and well-being.

Mental well-being refers to how you feel in general in life. How easy is it for you to deal with daily stresses and challenges?

If we have a higher sense of mental well-being, we are more likely to have high self-esteem and low levels of anxiety, depression, and stress.

But what can we do to influence these variables?

Physical activities, such as chair yoga, can be a source of enjoyment and happiness, according to a recent review by Sport England. They can boost our self-esteem and cognitive abilities. In addition, it reduces anxiety, depression, and stress.

We take time to sit quietly during yoga. We begin to pay attention to how our bodies feel and to our breathing. We try to keep our minds focused on observing our breath and body in the present moment.

As we begin to make gentle movements with our bodies, we focus our attention—as much as possible—on the experience of moving.

By focusing on the body and breath, we can slow down our thinking process. The mind begins to calm down, and our stress levels begin to decrease.

This can make us feel more peaceful and relaxed, as well as improve our overall quality of life.

9. During a busy day, take short energizing breaks.

You may notice that you begin to lose energy during the course of a busy day. After a few hours of nonstop work on the same thing, you become less productive. As a result, we are less energized and focused on our work.

You can help regulate your energy levels and be more efficient at work by incorporating very short breaks into your busy day.

Chair yoga provides a gentle way to break up long periods of inactivity. This gives us more energy and allows us to focus better on our work afterward.

The great thing about chair yoga is that no extra time is required to set up equipment or change your clothes. Removing some of the physical and mental obstacles to finding enough time to practice yoga.

All you have to do is take a few minutes out of your day to practice a chair yoga pose or sequence in your own chair!

As a result, it is easier to practice more frequently—even when you are short on time.

10. Develop yourself by learning a new skill.

As with learning any new skill, beginning to practice chair yoga as a beginner can be a fantastic opportunity for personal growth.

You'll learn to tune into your body, breath, and mind. Making different physical movements with your body can boost your confidence and self-esteem.

Sport England's recent review provides scientific evidence that learning and practicing exercises such as chair yoga can aid in the development of soft and social skills. Additionally, it will have a positive impact on your employment opportunities.

When you practice chair yoga with others, whether in a private class with a teacher or with a group of coworkers, it can help you form new social bonds and connections.

Chair Yoga Equipment Required

It's difficult to know what you really need to buy when you first start doing yoga. Because the yoga industry is constantly developing new clothing and equipment, you may believe that you must spend hundreds of dollars before entering a studio or class.

The good news is that you don't need much to get started. That being said, if you're starting an at-home practice or would prefer to buy yoga-specific clothing and equipment before your first class, here's what you need to know.

When practicing yoga, two types of equipment or gear are required. They are appropriate clothing as well as a yoga mat.

Clothing

Most yoga studios expect you to wear something to class, which should go without saying. However, you do not need a slew of printed yoga pants or designer clothing to be accepted by your peers. Here are some clothing options to consider.

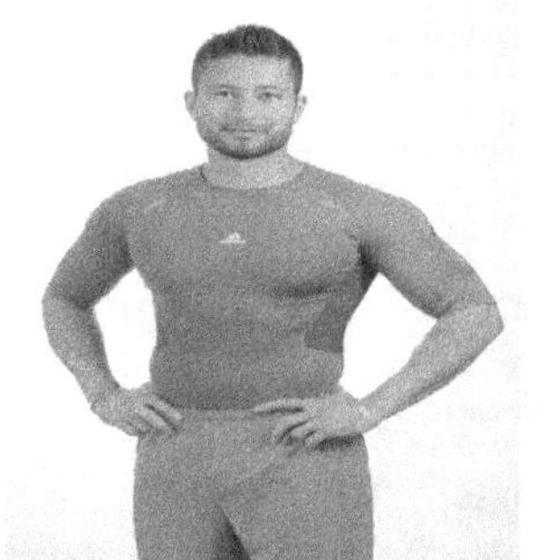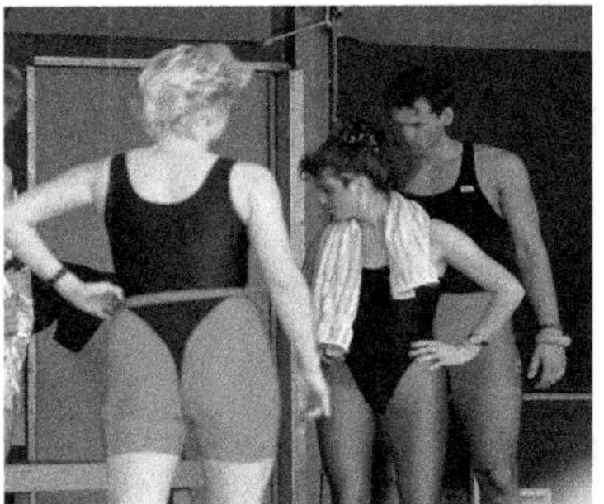

Yoga Pants: A few pairs of solid-color yoga pants in black, dark grey, navy, or brown can't go wrong. Alternatively, be daring and incorporate trendy prints or styles into your wardrobe. When you buy high-quality options, they can last for a long time.

Loose Pants: If you don't like tight pants, look for jogger-style pants or the popular harem-style pants with elastic around the ankles. These pants are stretchy and provide a little extra room, but the ankle elastic ensures that they stay in place throughout your practice.

Shorts: Shorts are a popular choice among men. They are also suitable for women, especially if you intend to try hot yoga. Look for form-fitting spandex shorts or looser shorts with connected tights underneath because some poses require you to position your legs in a way that looser, running-style shorts may leave you uncomfortably exposed.

Tops: It's critical to wear form-fitting tops so your shirt doesn't fly over your head during forward or backward bends. Wicking material is beneficial, especially if you sweat a lot or plan to attend a hot yoga class.

Cover-ups: Because yoga studios are sometimes kept cool, you may want to bring a light cover-up or sweater. Wear it until the class begins, and if you keep it near your mat, you can put it on before the final savasana.

Yoga is a low-impact activity, but a good sports bra can help keep your "girls" in place as you transition between poses, making your practice more comfortable.

Hair ties or headbands: If you have long hair, tie it back before class to keep stray locks out of your eyes and face. A simple hair tie or headband should suffice.

Socks for Yoga: To be clear, wearing yoga socks is not required to attend a class. In fact, doing yoga barefoot is preferable. If you can't bear the thought of walking around with bare feet, invest in a pair of yoga socks with bottom grips to keep your feet covered while maintaining good traction. Standard socks will not suffice, as you will end up slipping and sliding all over your mat.

Yoga clothing is now available almost anywhere. Though it's not uncommon to see yoga pants costing more than $100, don't feel obligated to spend that much money on just one pair. Several stores provide high-quality options for under $50. Purchase a few pairs of pants and tops and you'll be set for months.

Begin with comfortable, breathable athletic apparel you already own and supplement with mid-level basics if necessary.

The Yoga Mat

A yoga mat, also known as a sticky mat, is commonly used in gyms and yoga studios. This mat helps define your personal space while also providing traction for your hands and feet so you don't slip, especially if you're sweaty. It also adds some cushioning to a hard floor.

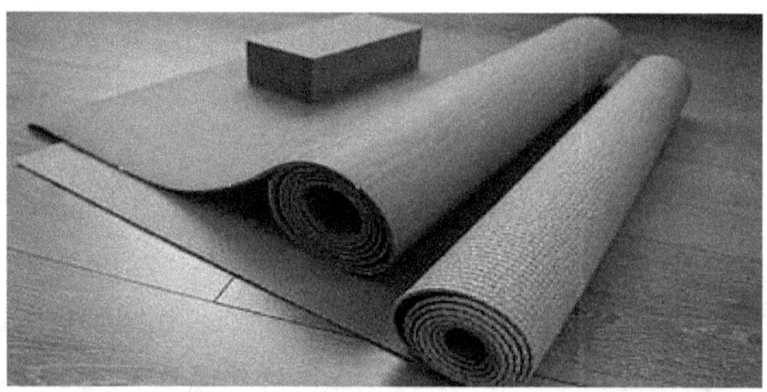

Most gyms provide mats, and studios rent them for a dollar or two per class. This is fine for your first few classes, but the disadvantage of these mats is that many people use them and you don't know how frequently they are cleaned. As a result, you should think about purchasing your own.

Premium yoga mats can be pricey, ranging from $80 to $120. A starter mat can also be found for as little as $20 at various retailers. Just keep in mind that if you buy a cheaper mat, you'll probably find yourself replacing it quickly if you use it frequently.

Determine which mat features are essential to you. Consider mat length, thickness, material, durability, comfort, traction, and even how to clean it. Then, based on your requirements, purchase a mat with positive reviews.

If you're serious about starting a yoga practice, your mat is one place where you should spend some money.

Yoga Equipment (Optional)

Yoga props are extremely beneficial to a new yoga practice. Props enable students to maintain the best alignment possible in a variety of poses as the body bends, twists, and open up. They also assist you in making the most of each pose while avoiding injury. 1

You should become acquainted with the props described below, but unless you are starting a home-based yoga practice, you do not need to purchase your own because they are almost always provided by studios and gyms.

Yoga Subscription Boxes That Work

Slings or Mat Bags

If you own your own yoga mat and are going to be lugging it back and forth to the studio on a regular basis, a mat bag or sling is a good investment. These accessories do exactly what they say: they allow you to sling your rolled mat over your shoulder without it unraveling.

Slings typically bind your mat in its rolled configuration with velcro straps and a connecting strap that can be thrown over your shoulder. They may also include additional storage pockets on occasion, but not always.

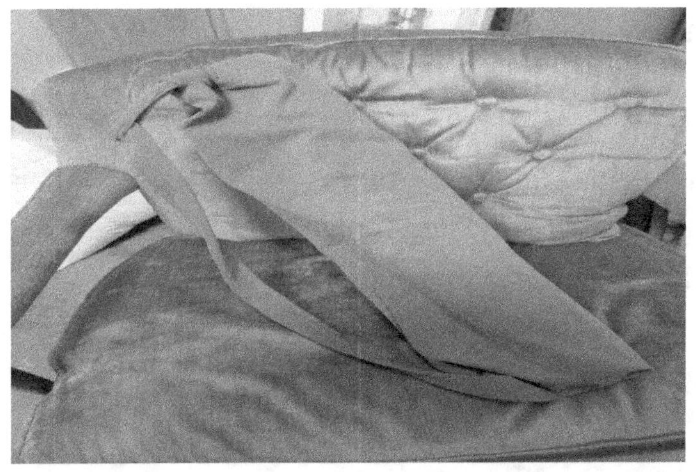

Bags, on the other hand, are typically divided into two types. One version employs velcro straps to secure your rolled mat against a larger gym bag. The other option is essentially a snap or zipper-closure bag designed specifically to hold your rolled mat.

Both styles offer additional storage for items such as clothing, wallets, and cell phones. It all comes down to personal preference and budget, as slings can cost as little as $10 while heavy-duty bags can cost well over $100.

Blankets Stacks of blankets are usually available in yoga studios for students to use during class. Folded blankets can be used to raise the hips in seated poses and to provide support in lying poses. So, at the start of class, grab one or two.

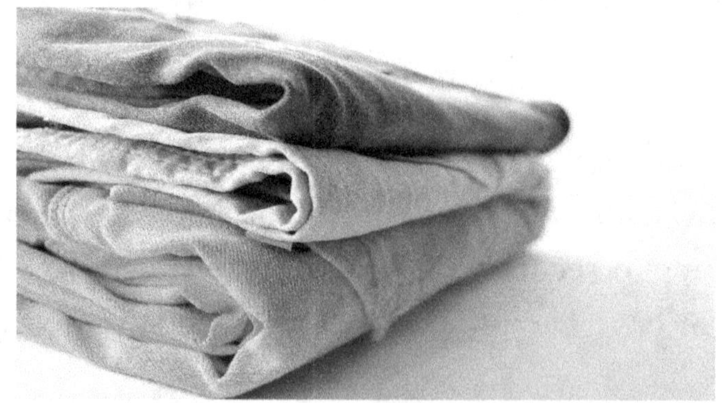

When sitting cross-legged, for example, you can elevate your hips above your knees by placing a blanket under your sit bones. Blankets are useful for a variety of purposes during class, and if it's cold outside, you can even use them to cover up during the final relaxation.

There's no reason to buy new blankets for home practice. Simply make use of what you already have around the house. If you don't have any extra blankets, you can frequently find them for as little as $13.

Blocks

Yoga blocks, like blankets, are used to make you more comfortable and to improve your alignment. Blocks are especially useful for standing poses that require your hands to be on the floor.

Blocks have the effect of "raising the floor" to meet your hands, as opposed to forcing the hands to come to the floor, potentially jeopardizing some aspect of the pose. They make it easier to maintain an open chest and a strong torso while avoiding misalignments such as:

1. Turning the chest toward the floor
2. The bending of the supporting knee
3. The torso's proclivity to "collapse"
4. Blocks can be useful in poses like Half Moon because many people lack the hamstring flexibility and core strength required to hold this position properly.

Yoga blocks are available in foam, wood, and cork. They can be rotated to stand at three different heights, making them extremely versatile. If you do a lot of yoga at home, getting a set of blocks for poses where both hands are reaching toward the ground is worthwhile. Blocks will be provided if you plan to attend classes.

The good news is that almost any block will suffice, so this is not an area where you should cut corners. However, slightly wider blocks (at least four inches wide) provide more stability. Several sizes and styles are available for under $10 each.

Straps

Yoga straps, also known as belts, come in handy when you need to hold onto your feet but can't reach them. The strap essentially serves as an arm extender.

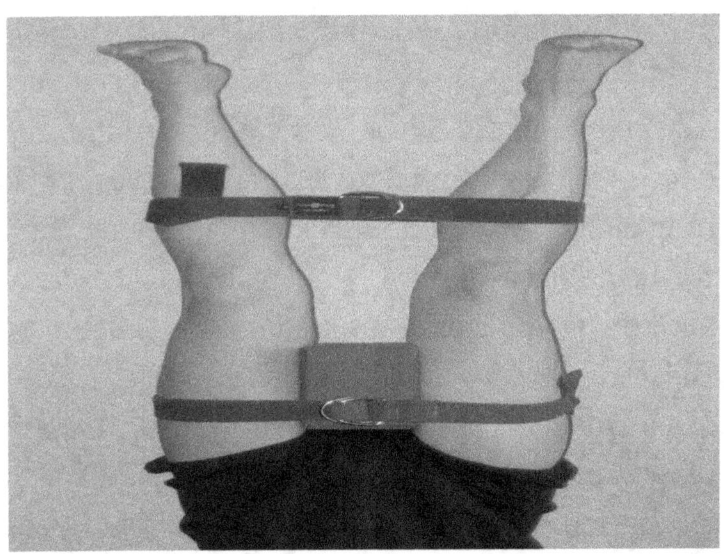

For example, if you can't reach your feet with your hands in Pascimottanasana (Seated Forward Bend), wrap the strap around the bottom of your feet and hold onto it to maintain a flat back instead of slumping forward.

Straps are also useful for poses in which you bind your hands behind your back (Marichyasana, for example). If your shoulders aren't flexible enough for the bind, you can use a strap to "connect" both hands without strain until you're able to progress to the full bind.

You most likely have something around the house that would work as a strap (such as a belt or even a towel), and yoga studios provide them for use during class. If you really want to buy your own, straps can be found for under $10.

Bolsters

Yoga students can put bolsters to use in a variety of ways. They can be used instead of a blanket stack to make seated and forward-bending poses more comfortable. When reclining, you can also place them under your knees or your back for support and passive stretching.

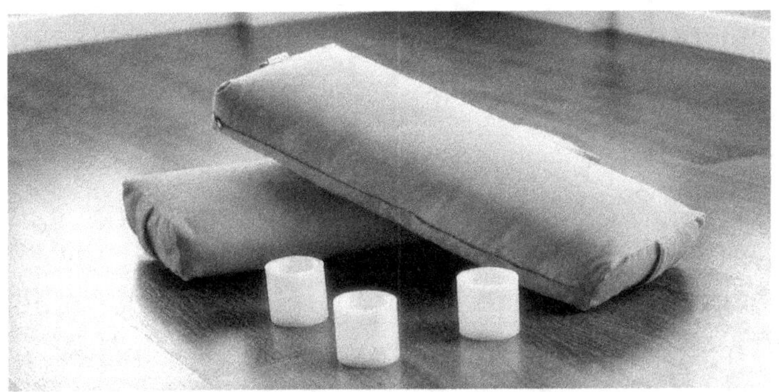

Bolsters come in handy, especially in restorative and prenatal yoga classes. The bolsters will be provided if you take this type of class. If you want to practice restorative yoga at home, it may be worthwhile to purchase your own bolster.

There are two types of bolsters: round and flat (more of a rectangular shape). Although flat bolsters are more ergonomic, round bolsters can be useful when you need more support or a deeper stretch. It all comes down to personal taste.

If possible, use both styles in class before deciding which one is best for your home practice. The prices range from $40 to $80, and the design options are both colorful and appealing.

Yoga wheels are a relatively new prop that is beginning to gain traction in the yoga studio. These wheels are approximately 12 inches in diameter and four inches in width.

When the wheel is upright, you can lie back on it or place a foot or hand on top to deepen stretches and increase flexibility, slowly rolling the wheel as you relax into the stretch. Wheels can also be used in more advanced practices to test stability or provide support.

While you are unlikely to require a yoga wheel as a beginner, you may want to consider purchasing one later on. The majority of wheels cost between $40 and $60.

12-Minute Chair Yoga Routines for Seniors

How do seniors practice chair yoga?

Here's a short routine with some recommended poses that my older students enjoy to help provide options. Remember that it's all about your comfort. At the start of each class, I remind students that we all have different physical makeups, live with different injuries and ranges of motion and that any posture that isn't working in their bodies should be skipped or modified.
In terms of chair yoga for seniors with music, I generally avoid music in my assisted living and nursing home sessions, but we frequently listen to some of their favorite tunes before and after class to build community and have some fun. Check out these chair exercises for seniors if you want to talk about more activities.

Are you ready to begin?

Make sure you have a chair with a flat back, either with or without arms. You are ready to go if you are in a wheelchair!

1. Reconnect with your breath

Spend a few moments or minutes connecting with your breath. Take note of the coolness of your breath as it enters your nostrils. Feel the warmth of your exhale. Simply breathe and be mindful of the qualities of your breath, perhaps noticing the expansion of your belly and ribs as you inhale and then letting go of the exhale. Breathing is the source of life.

2. Mountain stance

Work with mountain pose to develop a strong, foundational seat. Inhale and sit tall in your chair, feet hip-distance apart, feet on the ground, toes pointed forward (if you are able to).

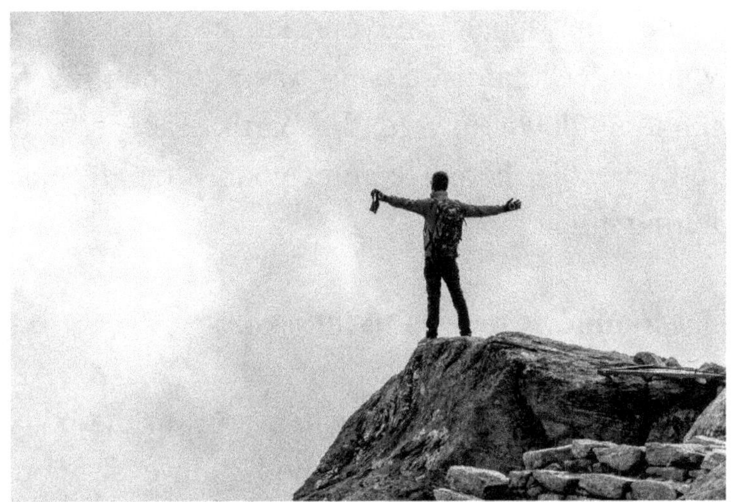

Shrug your shoulders toward your ears and draw the shoulders back and down your back as you continue to breathe comfortably. Take note of the opening across the collarbones.

Imagine a helium balloon tied to the top of your head on your next inhale, and lengthen your spine to sit up a little straighter.

Draw your belly button gently toward your spine to strengthen your core.

Place your hands on your lap or down along your sides, palms facing forward and fingers pointing down toward the earth. Take several full breaths here, feeling your strength and letting go.

3. **Shoulder shrugs and let's go.**

The following exercises will warm up the body and help us connect with the breath even more by tying the breath to movement.

Inhale and shrug your shoulders up toward your ears, then exhale and release. An audible exhale can be very refreshing and therapeutic at times!

Rep 3–5 times more.

At the conclusion of each exercise. Relax in your chair and take a few deep breaths in and out to relax and take in the effects of the exercise.

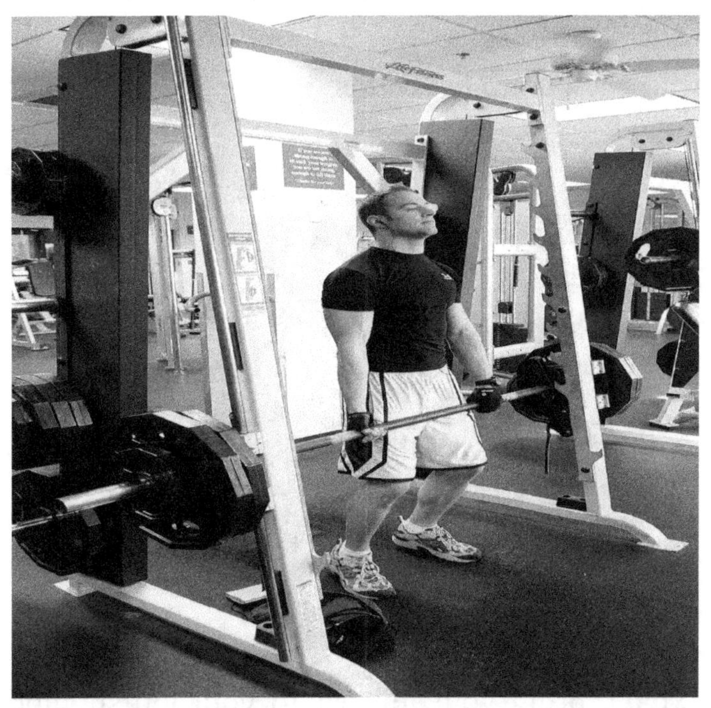

4. Gentle neck stretch from ear to shoulder

Sitting tall in your chair, roll your shoulders back and down your spine, gently squeezing the shoulder blade region.

Exhale and gently lower your right ear toward your right shoulder, starting at the center of your head. Hold for a few breaths, then inhale the head back up to the center.

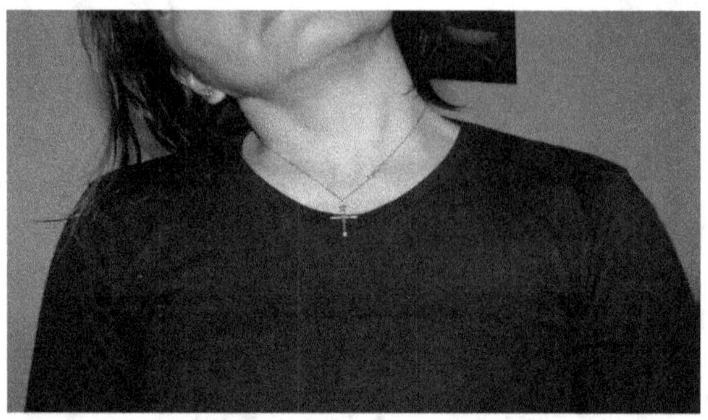

Exhale, bring your left ear to your left shoulder and breathe here for several rounds. Inhale and return to the center.

5. Front arm raises

Begin in mountain pose and extend your arms in front of you. (If this is too difficult on your shoulders, concentrate less on the arm lifting and lowering and instead work the movement gently and lower just above your lap.

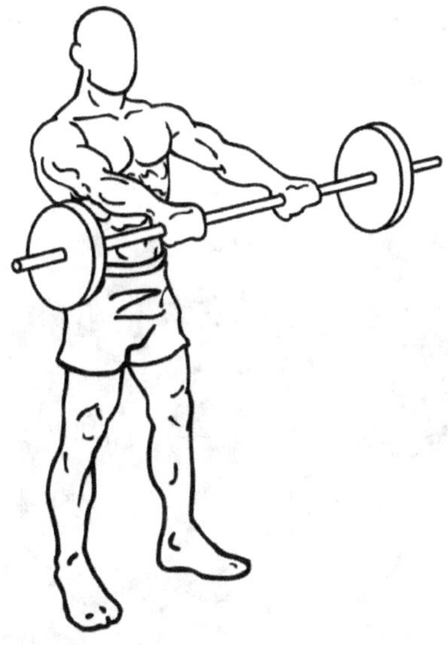

Inhale and raise your arms several inches, fingers pointing down.

Exhale and gently lower your arms back to your lap, fingers facing up.

Rep 3–5 times more.

6. **Side bend with cactus-like arms**

Inhale and bring your arms into a cactus or goal post position, drawing your shoulder blades together, beginning in a mountain pose.

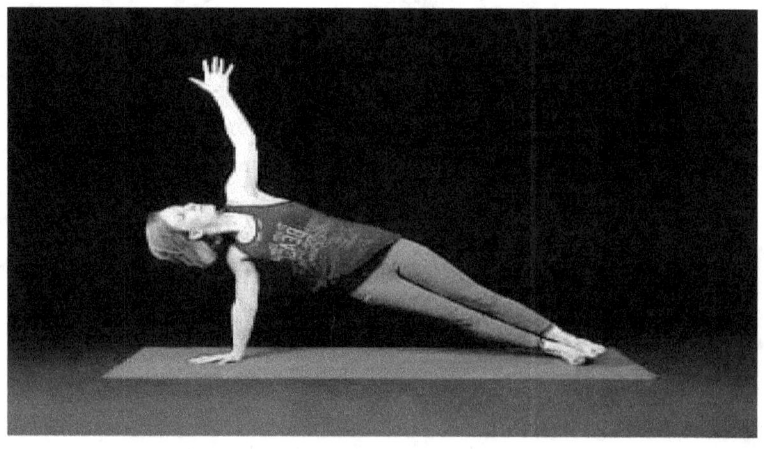

Exhale by gently bending your upper body to the left and taking a few deep breaths here.

Inhale and return to the center.

Exhale and gently bend your upper body to the right for a few rounds. Inhale and return to the center.

7. **Give the pot a good stir.**

Extend your legs a little wider and hold a ladle with both hands in front of your chest.

Visualize yourself gently stirring a pot. It could be as small as a saucepan or as large as a witch's cauldron!

Move your arms softly across your upper body, creating core mobility.

8. **Leg extension with a breath focus**

We'll now focus on engaging the lower body.

Inhale and lift your right leg from the mountain pose, possibly placing your right hand on your thigh just above your knee. On the inhale, notice how the quadriceps muscle engages. As you exhale, notice how it relaxes.

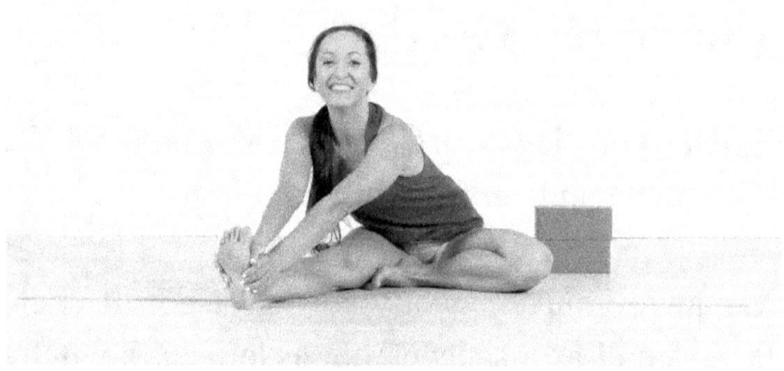

Work for 3 to 5 rounds here before resting and switching to the left side.

9. **Combination of toe raises and "pitter patter"**

We'll use a combination of toe raises and ankle dorsiflexion to draw the toes in toward the shin to balance muscle engagement in the calves and anterior tibia muscle in the shin area.

Beginning in mountain pose, exhale and lift your heels off the ground as if performing a toe raise.

Inhale and flex your ankle, pulling your toes toward your shin to activate the generally underactive muscles in the front lower region of the leg.

Work 5 to 10 finds of this combo before resting and observing the effect on your lower legs.

10. **Relaxation in a seated position.**

Returning to mountain pose, close your eyes, and just breathe. Take note of how your practice affects your mind and body.

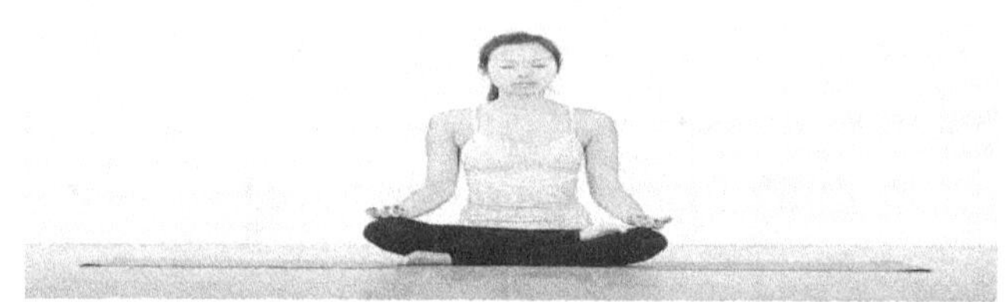

Feel your heart rate.

Allow your awareness to flow up and down your body like a continuous wave as you breathe.

Breathe here for a few rounds, then bring your hands together in front of your heart and thank yourself for committing to your practice.

Last Thoughts
Chair yoga for seniors and chair yoga for beginners make yoga benefits more accessible to a wider range of people.

Yoga for seniors has been shown to potentially reduce the risk of falls while also improving outlook, reducing pain, and improving osteoarthritis symptoms, among other benefits. Yoga for seniors is made safer and more confident by using a chair.

Traditional yoga poses, such as the mountain pose, can be used as a foundation posture in chair yoga routines for seniors.

Chair yoga should always feel comfortable and accessible to the individual. Students should be encouraged to avoid postures that do not feel good in their bodies and to always modify them to meet their individual requirements.

CHAPTER 2

Essential Stretching Exercises for Seniors to Do Every Day

It's never too late to start stretching.
Stretching may be your new best friend if you're a senior wanting to achieve greater independence, mobility, and flexibility (which may help you prevent falls and other accidents).

What about Flexibility?

Flexibility is a critical aspect of yoga practice. Yoga involves a wide range of physical postures, or asanas, which require varying degrees of flexibility in different parts of the body. In order to achieve these postures safely and effectively, it is essential to develop and maintain flexibility through regular practice. In this article, we will explore the role of flexibility in yoga, its benefits, and some tips for improving flexibility through yoga.

What is Flexibility in Yoga?

Flexibility refers to the ability of the muscles, tendons, and ligaments in the body to stretch and lengthen. In yoga, flexibility is important because it allows practitioners to move deeper into postures, improve alignment, and prevent injury. Each yoga posture requires a specific level of flexibility in different parts of the body. For example, a forward bend like Uttanasana requires flexibility in the hamstrings and lower back, while a backbend like Urdhva Dhanurasana requires flexibility in the shoulders and chest.

Benefits of Flexibility in Yoga

Improved Range of Motion: Flexibility in the muscles and joints allows for a greater range of motion. With greater range of motion, practitioners can achieve more challenging postures and deeper stretches.

Increased Strength: Flexibility in the muscles and joints also allows for greater strength. As the muscles become more flexible, they can contract and engage more effectively, leading to increased strength and stability in the body.

Reduced Risk of Injury: Flexibility helps to prevent injury by reducing tension in the muscles and ligaments. This allows the body to move more freely and with less strain, reducing the risk of muscle strain or tears.

Improved Posture: Flexibility can help to improve posture by lengthening and opening the muscles of the spine and shoulders. This can reduce tension in the neck and back and improve overall alignment.

Tips for Improving Flexibility in Yoga

Warm Up: Always begin your yoga practice with a gentle warm-up to prepare the body for stretching. This can include gentle movements like cat-cow, sun salutations, or simple stretches like seated forward folds.

Use Props: Yoga props like blocks, blankets, and straps can be used to modify postures and make them more accessible. Props can also help to support the body and allow for deeper stretches.

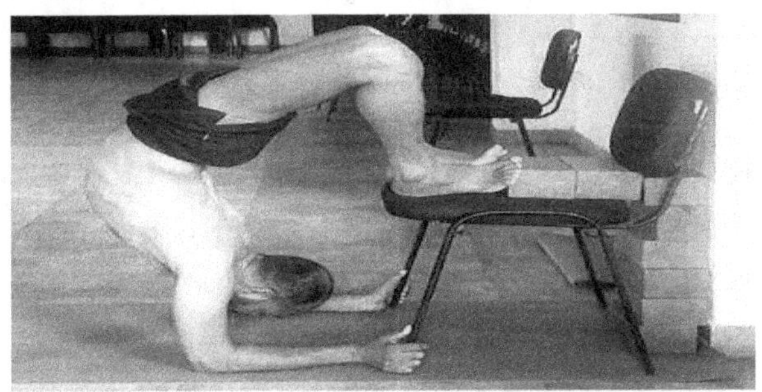

Focus on the Breath: The breath is an important tool for improving flexibility in yoga.

Focus on breathing deeply and slowly as you move through postures, and allow the breath to guide the movement of the body.

Practice Regularly: Consistency is key when it comes to improving flexibility in yoga. Practicing regularly, even for just a few minutes each day, can help to gradually increase flexibility and prevent the body from becoming stiff or tight.

Listen to Your Body: It is important to listen to your body and only push yourself as far as is comfortable. Overstretching can lead to injury, so always work within your limits and avoid pushing yourself too far too soon.

Flexibility is a crucial component of yoga practice. By improving flexibility through regular practice, practitioners can achieve deeper postures, improve alignment, and reduce the risk of injury. Incorporating the tips outlined above can help to improve flexibility and create a safe, effective yoga practice that supports overall health and wellbeing.

According to studies, flexibility in some joints declines by up to 50% with age. Because this decline occurs gradually over time, you may not even realize it. Then one day you attempt to grab for something or get up from the floor, and... ouch!

At this stage, many seniors resort to medicines, assistive medical devices, or even in-home caregivers to aid them with everyday tasks.

And, although these choices have their place in serious, advanced cases, what are the possibilities for persons who choose a more proactive approach?

Fortunately, research shows that stretching and range of motion exercises can help delay the loss of flexibility.

This is where our list of nine senior stretching exercises comes in.

These stretches consist of a combination of:

There are static stretches that promote flexibility and dynamic stretches that improve range of motion. They'll quickly help you feel more at ease in your own skin.

But first, let's define the distinction between static and dynamic stretches, because each has a purpose.

Stretching that is static
Static stretching is holding a stretch for 30 seconds or longer in order to lengthen a single muscle or group of muscles. Without bouncing or pushing/pulling, the stretch is constantly kept firmly.

Warming up is also essential before beginning static stretching, which we'll go into later.

Stretching in a Dynamic Environment

Dynamic stretching, like static stretching, is intended to stretch a set of muscles in a more dynamic manner.

It simply entails simulating real-world activities while stretching your muscles and getting your blood circulating.

Because it focuses on extending entirely through a natural action, dynamic stretching is good for enhancing your range of motion.

9 Essential Stretching Exercises for Seniors to Do Every Day

Try to execute these stretches every day, or as often as possible, to enhance your flexibility and mobility (essentially, your capacity to "move around").

Do a 5 to 10 minute warm up before stretching, including easy activities like walking in place and arm circles to get your muscles and joints warm.

1. Neck Stretch Side Neck Stretch

Because it is so basic, this is one of the greatest morning stretching exercises for seniors.

This neck side stretch will relieve any stress in your neck and tops of your shoulders caused by sleeping in the improper posture for an extended period of time or from not having enough pillow cushion at night.

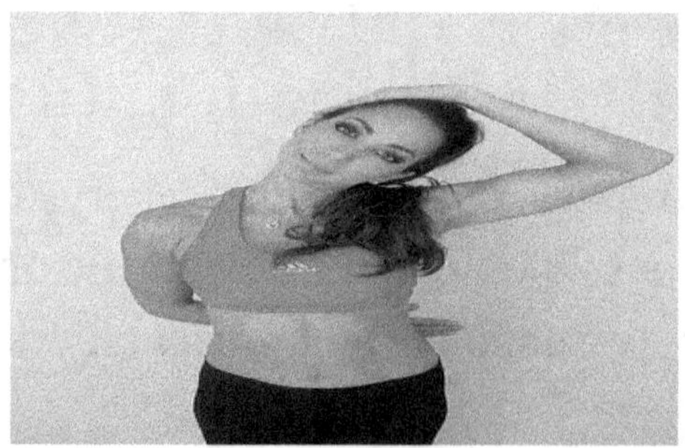

Begin by sitting up straight in a chair. Warm up your neck by gently leaning your head to one side, then the other.

Lift your right arm up and above your head, softly resting your palm on the left side.

Pull your head to the right slightly (very gently – in fact just placing your hand there may be enough weight to cause you to feel the stretch).

Hold for 20 to 30 seconds before repeating on the opposite side.

2. Hand Clasp Stretch Shoulder and Upper Back Stretch

Do you ever find it difficult to stand up straight because of a tight back? This is most likely due to your shoulders and upper back rounding forward when sitting.

Because the muscles are so used to being slumped, it might become difficult to stand up straight over time. This shoulder stretch will assist in loosening these muscles and improving spinal flexibility, allowing you to stand straight once again.

Begin by standing tall with your arms by your sides. Pull your shoulders back and clasp your fingers together by reaching behind you with both hands.
Hold it here if you already feel a stretch. Push your clasped hands away from your lower back and gently arc backward if you can.
Return to a tall stance and repeat.

3. Triceps Extension

This triceps stretch, which can be done standing or sitting, is excellent for increasing flexibility and mobility in the arms and upper back.

Lift your right arm up over your head, bending at the elbow, while sitting tall in a chair (or standing).
Reach your opposite arm up and grab your elbow, then slowly pull in the other way. A

gentle stretch should be felt through the back of your arm.

Hold for 20 to 30 seconds before switching arms.

4. Low Back Stretch

This back stretch is fantastic for increasing spine mobility and can even assist with rounded shoulders. It's also a little dynamic, which gets your blood pumping.

Begin by standing tall and placing your hands on your hips.
Arc backwards, staring up at the ceiling. Return to standing after about three seconds.
Rep 10 times more.

5. Taking a Position Quadriceps Flexion Quadriceps Flexion

This stretch is great for stretching the quadriceps muscle, which is located in the front of your thigh. This region is frequently shortened and tightened as a result of sitting or hunching forward, which can cause discomfort and aggravation of improper posture.

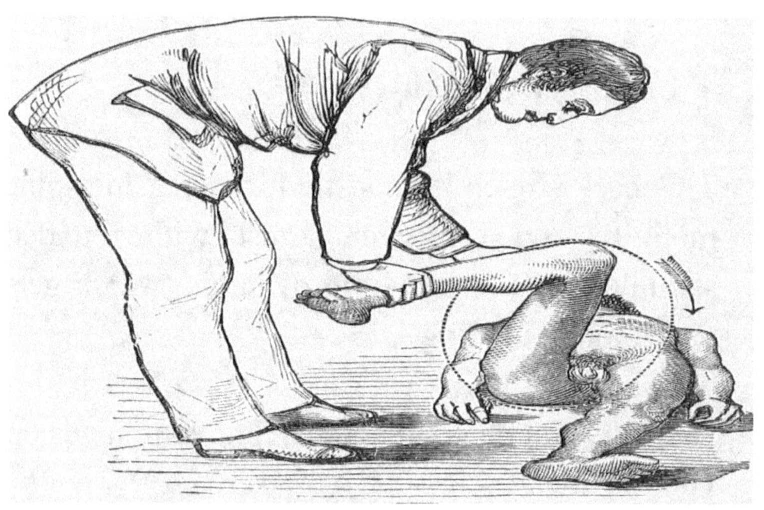

Begin by rising tall and balancing on the back of a chair or countertop with your free hand.
Bend your right knee slowly and hold your foot. You may already feel a stretch in the front of your thigh at this stage.
Hold this stretch for 30 seconds, then switch legs.

If you're having problems reaching your foot with your hand, as described above, consider using a yoga strap or band.

When it comes to keeping your balance, stiff and/or weak ankles are terrible news. Gaining more flexibility in this area creates a first line of protection against falls and stumbles.

6. **Sit tall and comfy on a robust chair.**
Extend your right leg in front of you while maintaining your left leg on the floor.
Begin rotating your right ankle 10 to 20 times clockwise and 10 to 20 times counter-clockwise.
Lower your leg and then repeat with the opposing leg.

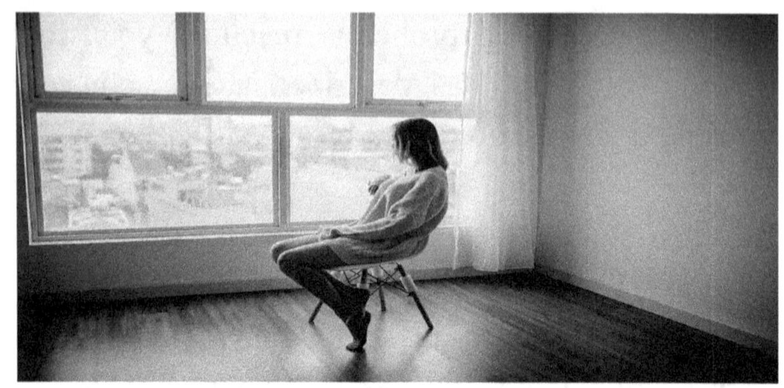

7. Sitting Hip Stretch
Hip Stretch While Sitting

Tight hips can make it difficult to do everyday tasks such as stepping out of a car or a bathtub. This hip stretch can assist develop hip flexibility, allowing you to move more freely.

Begin by sitting up straight in a firm chair.
Cross your right leg over your left, allowing your right ankle to rest on top of your left knee.
Let gravity draw your right hip toward the floor.
You may already feel a deep stretch in your hip.

To get a deeper stretch, softly press down on your right leg and knee.
Hold for 20 to 30 seconds before switching legs.

8. Cat-Cow Pose

The cat-cow position is a dynamic yoga stretch that is helpful for strengthening spine mobility and flexibility.

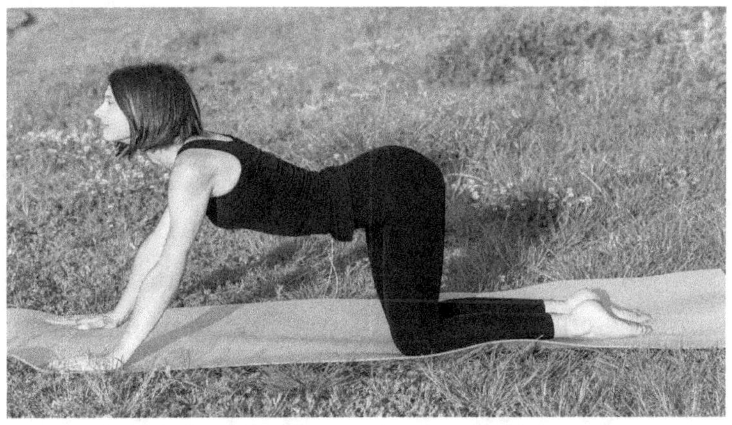

Begin on all fours on the floor. Place your hands firmly between your shoulders and your knees directly behind your hips. If your knees are sensitive, use extra cushioning (small cushions, towels, etc.).

Inhale while arching your spine and rising your head and chest toward the ceiling. Take a deep breath.

Now exhale while pushing your tummy in and lowering your head and neck (think like a startled Halloween cat).

Perform this exercise as many times as you desire, but at least 10 to 15 times.

9. Knee Tuck Stretch Hamstring and Low Back Stretch

This mild stretch focuses on the lower back and hamstrings, which can become tight and unpleasant as a result of extended sitting and/or bad posture.

Start this stretch by laying face up on your bed or the floor. Bend your right leg and bring it closer to your chest.

Maintain a flat back while you wrap your arms around your right knee (if you can't reach that far, consider grasping your trouser leg) and pull it toward you.

When you hold for 30 seconds, you should feel a tiny stretch in your low back, glutes, and hamstrings.

Rep with your opposite leg.

As you can see, even minor stretching may have great force.

If you want to develop greater freedom and control over your body as you age, I highly recommend incorporating these stretches into your daily routine and maybe enrolling in a regular fitness program.

Remember, a moving body continues moving.

Genie Stretching

Genie stretching, also known as knee stretching, is a stretching exercise that focuses on the muscles, tendons, and ligaments around the knee joint. It is a crucial part of any exercise routine, as it helps to improve the flexibility and range of motion of the knee joint, which can lead to a variety of benefits for overall health and fitness.

Benefits of Genie Stretching

1. *Improves flexibility and range of motion:* One of the most significant benefits of genie stretching is that it can help to improve the flexibility and range of motion of the knee joint. This can be particularly beneficial for individuals who engage in activities that require a lot of knee movement, such as running, jumping, or playing sports.

2. **Reduces the risk of injury:** By improving flexibility and range of motion, genie stretching can help to reduce the risk of injury to the knee

joint. Tight muscles, tendons, and ligaments can put increased stress on the knee joint during movement, increasing the risk of strain or tear. Stretching helps to loosen these structures, reducing the likelihood of injury.

3. **Eases knee pain:** Stretching can also help to ease knee pain by reducing tension in the muscles and ligaments surrounding the joint. This can be particularly beneficial for individuals with knee injuries, such as sprains or strains, as well as those with chronic knee pain due to conditions like arthritis.

4. **Enhances athletic performance**: By improving flexibility and range of motion, genie stretching can also help to enhance athletic performance. Athletes who have greater flexibility and range of motion in their knee joint may be able to move more easily and with greater agility, improving their overall performance on the field or court.

4. **Reduces muscle soreness:** Stretching after exercise can also help to reduce muscle soreness, which is particularly beneficial for individuals who engage in high-intensity activities that put a lot of strain on the knee joint, such as running or weightlifting.

How to perform Genie Stretching:

- Sit on the floor with your legs straight out in front of you.

- Bend your right knee and bring your foot towards your buttocks.

- Place your left hand on your right knee and gently pull it towards your left shoulder.

- Hold the stretch for 15-30 seconds, then release.

Repeat on the other side.

- For an additional stretch, cross your legs and place your right ankle over your left knee.

- Gently push down on your right knee to stretch the muscles and ligaments around your knee joint.

- Hold the stretch for 15-30 seconds, then release.

Repeat on the other side.

Genie stretching is an excellent way to improve flexibility, range of motion, and overall knee joint health. By regularly incorporating genue stretching into your exercise routine, you can reap the many benefits of this simple yet effective exercise, including reduced risk of injury, improved athletic performance, and reduced muscle soreness. So, take the time to stretch your knees and enjoy the benefits of a healthier, more mobile body.

CHAPTER 3

Basic and Core Strength Exercises

Basic and core strength exercises are an essential part of any man's fitness routine. Not only do they build strength and muscle mass, but they also help to improve posture, balance, and overall physical performance. In this article, we will explore some of the best basic and core strength exercises for men, their benefits, and tips for incorporating them into a workout routine.

Basic Strength Exercises for Men

Squats: Squats are one of the most effective exercises for building lower body strength. They work the quads, hamstrings, glutes, and calves, as well as the core and lower back. To perform a squat, stand with your feet shoulder-width apart, keeping your back straight and core engaged. Bend your knees and lower your hips down and back as if sitting in a chair, keeping your weight in your heels. Return to standing position and repeat.

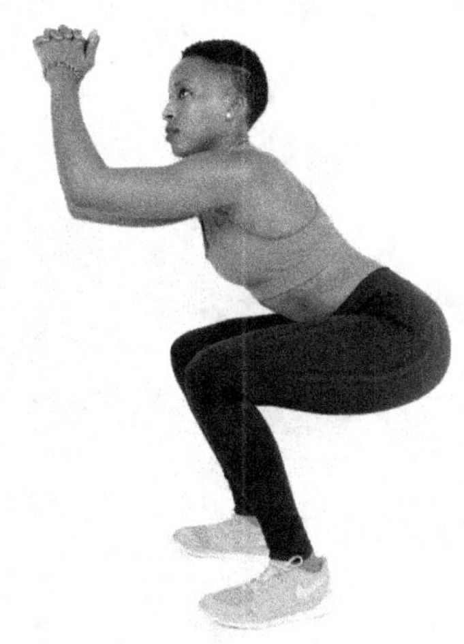

Deadlifts: Deadlifts are another great exercise for building overall strength, particularly in the legs, back, and core. To perform a deadlift, stand with your feet shoulder-width apart, keeping your back straight and core engaged. Hold a barbell or dumbbells in front of your thighs, then bend at the hips and knees, lowering the weights to the ground. Return to standing position and repeat.

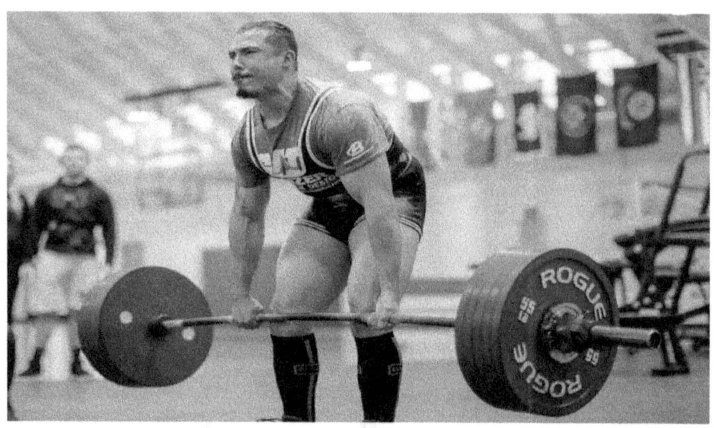

Push-Ups: Push-ups are a classic exercise that targets the chest, shoulders, triceps, and core. To perform a push-up, start in a plank position with your hands slightly wider than shoulder-width apart. Lower your body down towards the ground, keeping your elbows close to your body, then push back up to plank position.

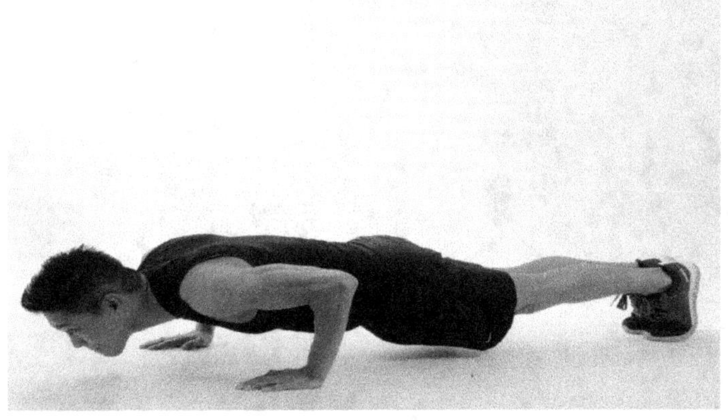

Pull-Ups: Pull-ups are a challenging exercise that targets the back, biceps, and shoulders. To perform a pull-up, grip a pull-up bar with your hands slightly wider than shoulder-width apart. Hang from the bar with your arms fully extended, then pull your body up towards the bar, keeping your elbows close to your body. Lower back down to starting position and repeat.

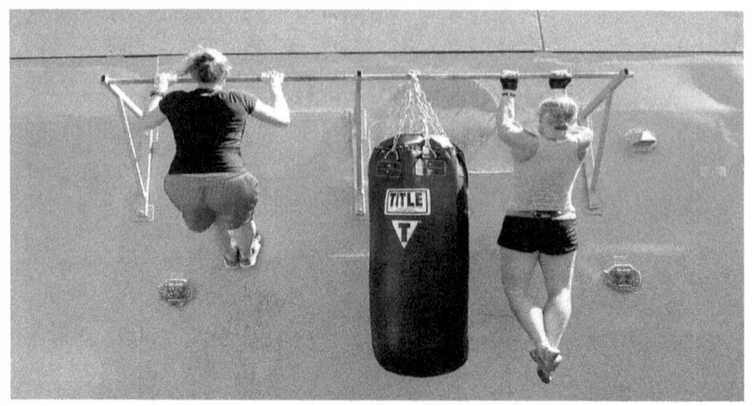

Core Strength Exercises for Men

Planks: Planks are a simple but effective exercise for building core strength. To perform a plank, start in a push-up position, then lower down onto your forearms. Keep your body in a straight line from head to heels, engaging your core muscles to hold the position for as long as possible.

Crunches: Crunches target the rectus abdominis, or "six-pack" muscles, as well as the obliques. To perform a crunch, lie on your back with your knees bent and feet flat on the ground.

Place your hands behind your head, then lift your head and shoulders off the ground, squeezing your abs at the top of the movement.

Russian Twists: Russian twists are a great exercise for building rotational strength and targeting the oblique muscles. To perform a Russian twist, sit on the ground with your knees bent and feet flat on the ground. Lean back slightly and lift your feet off the ground, balancing on your sit bones. Hold a weight or medicine ball in front of your chest, then rotate your torso from side to side, tapping the weight on the ground each time.

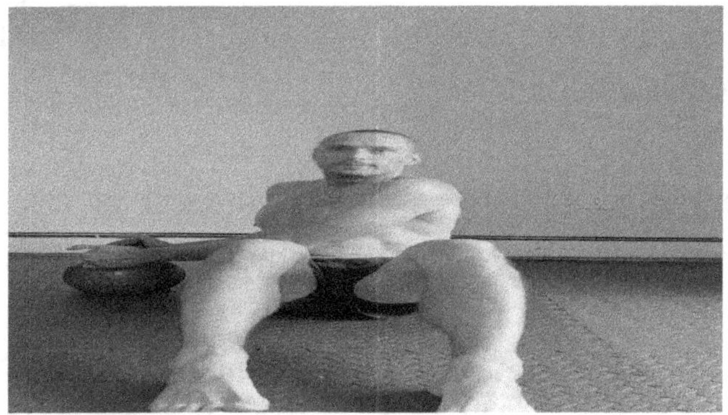

Leg Raises: Leg raises target the lower abs and hip flexors. To perform a leg raise, lie on your back with your hands by your sides. Lift your legs straight up towards the ceiling, keeping them together and your core engaged. Slowly lower your legs back down to starting position, then repeat.

Tips for Incorporating Basic and Core Strength Exercises into a Workout Routine

Start with the Basics: If you are new to strength training, start with the basic exercises outlined above and focus on perfecting your form before adding weight or increasing intensity.

Core training is an important aspect of overall fitness, as it helps to strengthen the muscles in the torso and pelvis, improving stability, balance, and posture. A strong core can also prevent back pain and improve athletic performance. In this article, we will explore some basic core training exercises that can boost your health and well-being.

Bridges: Bridges target the muscles in the lower back, glutes, and hamstrings. To perform a bridge, lie on your back with your knees bent and feet flat on the ground. Lift your hips up towards the ceiling, squeezing your glutes at the top of the movement. Lower back down to starting position and repeat. Bridges can be modified by adding a weight or performing single-leg bridges.

Dead Bugs: Dead bugs are a great exercise for improving coordination and stability while targeting the core muscles. To perform a dead bug, lie on your back with your arms extended towards the ceiling and your knees bent at a 90-degree angle. Lower one arm and the opposite leg towards the ground, then return to starting position and repeat on the other side.

Bird Dogs: Bird dogs are another exercise that improves coordination and stability while targeting the core muscles. To perform a bird dog, start on your hands and knees with your wrists under your shoulders and your knees under your hips. Extend one arm and the opposite leg straight out, then return to starting position and repeat on the other side.

Russian Twists: Russian twists are a great exercise for building rotational strength and targeting the oblique muscles. To perform a Russian twist, sit on the ground with your knees bent and feet flat on the ground. Lean back slightly and lift your feet off the ground, balancing on your sit bones. Hold a weight or medicine ball in front of your chest, then rotate your torso from side to side, tapping the weight on the ground each time.

Flutter Kicks: Flutter kicks are an effective exercise for targeting the lower abs and hip flexors. To perform flutter kicks, lie on your back with your legs extended straight out. Lift your legs off the ground and alternate kicking up and down in a quick, controlled motion.

Tips for Incorporating Core Training into Your Workout Routine

Start with the Basics: If you are new to core training, start with the basic exercises outlined above and focus on perfecting your form before adding weight or increasing intensity.

Mix it Up: Vary your core training exercises to prevent boredom and ensure that you are targeting all areas of your core.

Focus on Quality over Quantity: It is better to perform a few reps of each exercise with good form than to do many reps with poor form.

Incorporate Core Training into Your Overall Fitness Routine: Core training should be just one component of a well-rounded fitness routine that includes cardio, strength training, and flexibility exercises.

In conclusion, core training is an essential aspect of overall fitness that can boost your health and well-being. By incorporating basic core training exercises into your workout routine, you can strengthen your core muscles, improve your stability and balance, and prevent back pain. Remember to start with the basics, mix up your exercises, focus on quality over quantity, and incorporate core training into your overall fitness routine for optimal results.

Here are some tips on how to train the core in chair yoga:

Start with basic breathing exercises: Before you begin any physical activity, it's important to warm up your body and focus your mind. Start with some basic breathing exercises to help you relax and prepare for your yoga practice. Sit comfortably in your chair, with your feet flat on the ground and your hands resting on your knees. Take a deep breath in through your nose, filling your lungs completely, and then exhale slowly through your mouth. Repeat this several times, focusing on your breath and allowing your body to relax.

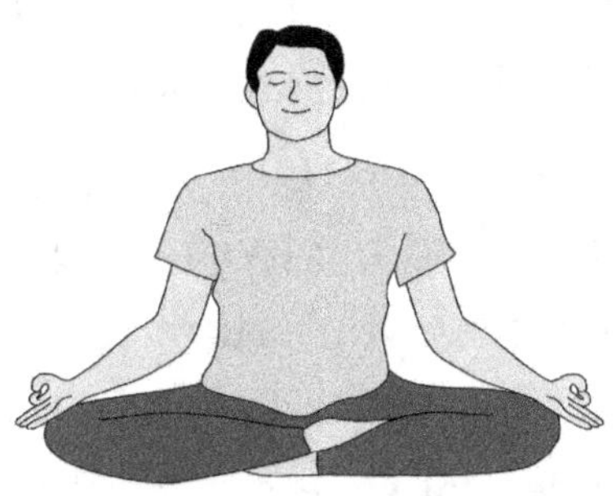

Engage your core muscles: To engage your core muscles, start by sitting up straight in your chair, with your feet flat on the ground and your hands resting on your thighs. Draw your navel in towards your spine, and then lift your ribcage up away from your hips. You should feel a gentle contraction in your abdominal muscles, as if you were trying to pull your belly button in towards your spine. Hold this contraction for a few seconds, and then release.

Practice seated twists: Seated twists are a great way to strengthen your core muscles and improve your spinal flexibility. Start by sitting up straight in your chair, with your feet flat on the ground and your hands resting on your thighs. Inhale deeply, and then as you exhale, twist your torso to the right, using your hands to help you turn. Hold the twist for a few seconds, and then inhale as you return to center. Repeat the twist to the left side, and then continue alternating sides for several repetitions.

Do seated leg lifts: Seated leg lifts are a great way to strengthen your lower abdominal muscles and improve your balance. Start by sitting up straight in your chair, with your feet flat on the ground and your hands resting on your thighs. Lift one foot off the ground, keeping your knee bent and your foot flexed. Hold the lift for a few seconds, and then lower your foot back down. Repeat on the other side, and then continue alternating sides for several repetitions.

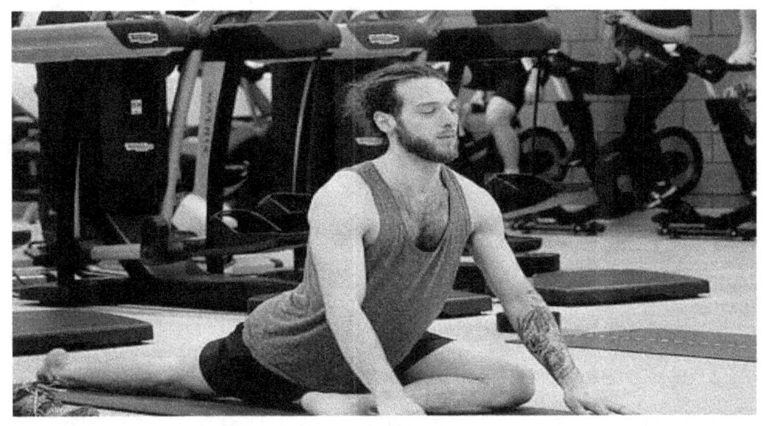

Try seated planks: Seated planks are a modified version of the traditional plank exercise, and they're a great way to strengthen your entire core. Start by sitting up straight in your chair, with your feet flat on the ground and your hands resting on your thighs. Lean forward slightly, and then place your hands on the armrests of your chair. Press down through your hands and lift your hips up, coming into a plank position. Hold the plank for a few seconds, and then lower your hips back down. Repeat for several repetitions.

Cool down with relaxation: After you've completed your core training exercises, it's important to take a few minutes to cool down and relax. Sit comfortably in your chair, with your feet flat on the ground and your hands resting on your thighs. Close your eyes and take a few deep breaths, allowing your body to relax and release any tension. Focus on the sensation of your breath moving in and out of your body, and allow yourself to fully unwind.

In conclusion, training your core in chair yoga is a great way to improve your balance, flexibility, and posture. By incorporating these exercises into your regular yoga.

Exercises that will improve your health

Sitting exercise

Sitting exercise is an excellent way to stay active and maintain good physical health, especially if you have a sedentary lifestyle or a job that requires you to sit for extended periods of time. With sitting exercises, you can engage your muscles, improve your flexibility, and enhance your overall well-being without having to leave your seat. In this article, we'll discuss some of the most effective sitting exercises that you can do to stay healthy and fit.

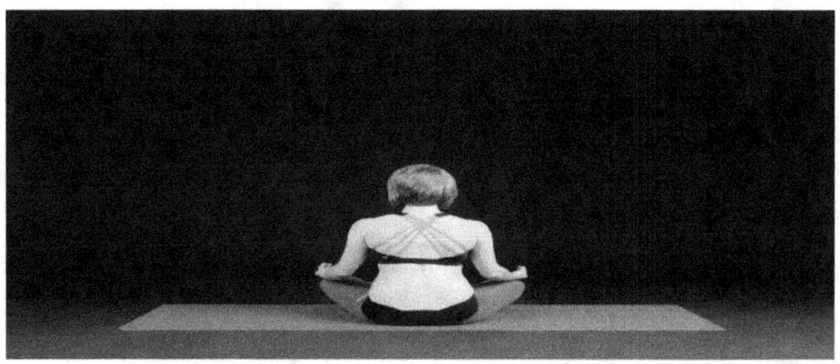

Seated Marching

Seated marching is an excellent exercise that can help to improve circulation, strengthen leg muscles, and increase range of motion. To perform this exercise, sit upright in your chair with your feet flat on the ground. Lift one knee up towards your chest, and then lower it back down. Repeat with the other leg, and continue alternating for 30 seconds to 1 minute.

Seated Leg Extensions

Seated leg extensions are a great way to tone your leg muscles and improve your balance. To perform this exercise, sit upright in your chair with your feet flat on the ground. Slowly extend one leg out in front of you, keeping it straight and parallel to the ground. Hold for a few seconds, and then lower your leg back down. Repeat with the other leg, and continue alternating for 30 seconds to 1 minute.

Seated Twist

Seated twists are an excellent way to improve spinal mobility and increase core strength. To perform this exercise, sit upright in your chair with your feet flat on the ground. Place your left hand on the outside of your right knee, and then slowly twist your torso to the right. Hold for a few seconds, and then return to center. Repeat on the other side, and continue alternating for 30 seconds to 1 minute.

Shoulder Shrugs

Shoulder shrugs are a simple yet effective exercise that can help to relieve tension in your neck and shoulders. To perform this exercise, sit upright in your chair with your feet flat on the ground. Slowly raise your shoulders up towards your ears, hold for a few seconds, and then release. Repeat for 10 to 15 repetitions.

Seated Cat-Cow Stretch

Seated cat-cow stretch is a yoga-inspired exercise that can help to improve spinal mobility and relieve tension in your back muscles. To perform this exercise, sit upright in your chair with your feet flat on the ground. Place your hands on your knees, and then arch your spine upwards, lifting your chest towards the ceiling. Hold for a few seconds, and then round your spine downwards, tucking your chin towards your chest. Repeat for 10 to 15 repetitions.

Seated Hip Stretch

Seated hip stretch is an excellent exercise that can help to improve hip flexibility and relieve tension in your lower back. To perform this exercise, sit upright in your chair with your feet flat on the ground. Cross your right ankle over your left knee, and then gently press your right knee down towards the ground. Hold for a few seconds, and then release. Repeat on the other side, and continue alternating for 30 seconds to 1 minute.

Seated Push-Ups

Seated push-ups are a great way to build upper body strength and improve core stability. To perform this exercise, sit upright in your chair with your feet flat on the ground. Place your hands on the armrests of your chair, and then slowly push yourself up, lifting your hips off the seat. Hold for a few seconds, and then lower yourself back down. Repeat for 10 to 15 repetitions.

In conclusion, sitting exercise is a great way to stay active and improve your physical health, even if you have limited mobility or access to a gym.

Important things to do before exercise

When it comes to exercise, many people focus solely on the main activity and forget about the importance of a proper warm-up, cool-down, and supporting exercises like mat and weight exercises. These elements are essential to preventing injury, improving performance, and promoting overall fitness. In this article, we'll delve into the specifics of warming up, mat and weight exercises, cooling down, and standing exercises.

Warming up

Before diving into any exercise, it's important to warm up your muscles, ligaments, and joints. Warming up helps prepare your body for physical activity, improves blood flow, and increases the range of motion of your joints. This can help reduce the risk of injury and improve your overall performance during your workout.

A good warm-up should last anywhere from 5 to 15 minutes and should include light cardiovascular exercises like jogging or jumping jacks, as well as dynamic stretching. Dynamic stretching involves moving your muscles through a range of motion, such as lunges or arm circles, rather than holding a stretch for an extended period of time. This type of stretching helps to loosen up your muscles and prepare them for more strenuous activity.

Mat and weight exercises

Mat and weight exercises are an excellent way to improve strength, balance, and flexibility. Mat exercises are typically done on the ground and focus on bodyweight movements such as planks, crunches, and push-ups. These exercises are great for developing core strength and improving posture.

Weight exercises, on the other hand, involve lifting weights or resistance bands to increase muscle strength and size. Weight exercises can be done using free weights or machines, and can target specific muscle groups such as the biceps, triceps, or quadriceps.

When performing mat or weight exercises, it's important to use proper form to prevent injury and maximize the benefits of the exercise. Start with lighter weights or bodyweight movements and gradually increase the resistance or difficulty level as your strength and technique improve.

Cooling down

After completing your workout, it's important to cool down to gradually bring your heart rate and breathing back to normal. A cool-down should last about 5 to 10 minutes and should include light cardio exercises like walking or cycling, as well as static stretching.

Static stretching involves holding a stretch for an extended period of time to improve flexibility and reduce muscle tension. This type of stretching is different from dynamic stretching and should be done when your muscles are already warmed up.

Standing exercises

Standing exercises are any exercises that are performed while standing, such as squats, lunges, and calf raises. These exercises help improve balance, coordination, and lower body strength.

Standing exercises can be done with or without weights and can be modified to suit different fitness levels. For example, beginners may start with bodyweight squats, while more advanced exercisers may use a barbell or kettlebell to add resistance.

When performing standing exercises, it's important to maintain proper form to prevent injury and maximize the benefits of the exercise. This includes keeping your knees in line with your toes during squats and lunges, and keeping your back straight during deadlifts.

In conclusion, warming up, mat and weight exercises, cooling down, and standing exercises are all important elements of a well-rounded fitness routine. By incorporating these exercises into your workout, you can improve your overall fitness, prevent injury, and achieve your fitness goals

Weekly schedule of chair yoga exercises

Monday: Warm-Up

Begin your week with a gentle warm-up to help prepare your body for the week ahead. Start by sitting upright in your chair with your feet flat on the ground and your hands resting on your thighs. Take a few deep breaths, inhaling through your nose and exhaling through your mouth.

Next, slowly raise your arms up to shoulder height, reaching towards the ceiling. Hold for a few breaths, then slowly lower your arms back down to your thighs. Repeat this movement 5-10 times, focusing on your breath and the sensations in your body.

Finally, gently twist your torso to the right, placing your left hand on the outside of your right thigh and your right hand on the armrest of your chair. Hold for a few breaths, then release and repeat on the other side. This will help to release tension in your spine and improve your flexibility.

Tuesday: Core Strength

On Tuesday, focus on building strength in your core muscles with these simple chair yoga exercises. Begin by sitting upright in your chair with your feet flat on the ground and your hands resting on your thighs. Take a few deep breaths, inhaling through your nose and exhaling through your mouth.

Next, bring your hands together in front of your chest and twist your torso to the right, bringing your left elbow towards your right knee. Hold for a few breaths, then release and repeat on the other side. This will help to strengthen your oblique muscles and improve your balance.

Finally, lift your feet off the ground and hold them there for a few seconds, engaging your core muscles to maintain your balance. Lower your feet back down and repeat 5-10 times, focusing on your breath and the sensations in your body.

Wednesday: Upper Body Stretch

On Wednesday, focus on stretching your upper body with these simple chair yoga exercises. Begin by sitting upright in your chair with your feet flat on the ground and your hands resting on your thighs. Take a few deep breaths, inhaling through your nose and exhaling through your mouth.

Next, reach your arms up towards the ceiling, clasping your hands together if possible. Hold for a few breaths, then slowly lean to the right, stretching the left side of your body. Hold for a few breaths, then release and repeat on the other side.

Finally, interlace your fingers behind your back and gently lift your arms up, stretching your chest and shoulders. Hold for a few breaths, then release and repeat 5-10 times, focusing on your breath and the sensations in your body.

Thursday: Balance Practice

On Thursday, focus on improving your balance with these simple chair yoga exercises. Begin by sitting upright in your chair with your feet flat on the ground and your hands resting on your thighs. Take a few deep breaths, inhaling through your nose and exhaling through your mouth.

Next, lift your right foot off the ground and balance on your left foot for a few seconds. Lower your right foot back down and repeat on the other side. This will help to improve your balance and stability.

Finally, practice a tree pose by lifting your right foot off the ground and placing it on your left inner thigh. Rest your hands on your thighs and hold for a few breaths, then release and repeat on the other side. This will help to improve your balance and focus.

Friday: Relaxation

On Friday, focus on relaxation and stress

CHAPTER 4

Strength Training Exercise for Elderly in 20 Minutes

Being active becomes increasingly vital as you get older. Frequent exercise can help you gain muscle mass, manage sickness or pain symptoms, promote independent living, and lower your risk of developing cardiovascular or neurological disorders. 1

This workout is specifically developed for seniors and contains movements that engage all of the major muscle groups throughout the body. This workout may be done at home or at a fitness club, whichever is most pleasurable and convenient for you. There is no need for specialized equipment. You'll also note that some of the exercises assist you enhance or maintain functional stability and balance, ensuring that daily tasks stay accessible as you age.

Precautions and Security

Before beginning this or any fitness program, consult with your healthcare professional to ensure that it is safe for you. Your clinician may recommend changes to improve your health.

Secondly, you'll want to select a place where you can do the exercises comfortably. Check that you can fully stretch your arms and move about without collapsing against any furniture or walls. Remove any little area rugs that might cause you to slip or trip. You can use a yoga mat for the floor exercises if you have one.

Finally, remember to work within your capabilities. There's no need to overwork oneself, especially when you're just getting started. It is acceptable to feel your body working and to expect some amount of difficulty, but you should not experience pain.

Yoga is a form of exercise that has been practiced for centuries. It has been found to have numerous benefits, both physical and mental. Chair yoga is a modified form of yoga that is suitable for individuals who have limited mobility or cannot perform traditional yoga poses due to physical limitations. Chair yoga can be done while sitting in a chair, making it accessible to individuals of all ages and fitness levels. In this chapter, we will explore the training plans for chair yoga.

The first step in designing a chair yoga training plan is to assess the needs of the individuals who will be participating in the program. This assessment should include an evaluation of the participants' physical abilities and any limitations they may have. This can be done through a questionnaire or a physical assessment.

Once the assessment is complete, the next step is to develop a series of chair yoga poses that are appropriate for the participants' needs. These poses should be tailored to each individual's level of ability and should include modifications for those who may need them.

When designing a chair yoga training plan, it is important to consider the overall goals of the program. For example, if the goal is to improve flexibility, the program should include a series of poses that focus on stretching and increasing range of motion. If the goal is to reduce stress and promote relaxation, the program should include poses that encourage deep breathing and meditation.

In addition to poses, the chair yoga training plan should also include a warm-up and cool-down period. The warm-up period should include gentle stretches and movements to prepare the body for the more challenging poses that will follow. The cool-down period should include poses that promote relaxation and reduce stress.

When designing a chair yoga training plan, it is important to consider the frequency and duration of the sessions. For beginners, it is recommended to start with shorter sessions and gradually increase the duration as their abilities improve. Ideally, participants should engage in chair yoga at least two to three times a week for optimal results.

It is also important to consider the environment in which the chair yoga sessions will take place. The space should be quiet, well-lit, and free of distractions. Participants should wear comfortable clothing and have access to a sturdy chair that is appropriate for their size and needs.

When teaching chair yoga, it is important to use clear and concise language to guide participants through the poses. It may also be helpful to provide visual aids or demonstrations to help participants better understand the poses.

As participants progress in their chair yoga practice, it may be beneficial to introduce more challenging poses and sequences. This can help to keep the practice interesting and engaging, while also providing opportunities for continued growth and development.

Chair Yoga Training Plan

Chair yoga is a valuable form of exercise that is accessible to individuals of all ages and fitness levels. When designing a chair yoga training plan, it is important to assess the needs of the participants, develop a series of poses and sequences that are appropriate for their abilities, and consider the overall goals of the program. With proper planning and instruction, chair yoga can provide numerous physical and mental benefits for those who participate.

Overview

Time allotted: 25 minutes (5-minute warm-up, 15 minutes strength training, 5-minute cool-down)

Beginning to intermediate level

Dumbbells or portable weights are required (3 to 5 pounds to start, 8 to 10 pounds as you get stronger). If you don't have any weights, try using household items like water bottles or soup cans.

What to Expect: If you're a newbie, perform the exercises with no weight at all at first. Simply concentrate on mastering the exercises with proper technique. Once you've mastered each technique, add dumbbells (or another kind of resistance) to the workouts that call for them.

A Beginner's Guide to Strengthening

5 minutes of warm-up
Warming up is key. Warming up dilates your blood vessels, allowing more oxygen to reach your muscles. A warm-up also gradually elevates your heart rate, reducing stress on your heart. 2

Do the following four warm-up movements for one minute each. Try not to pause between movements, but pause for a few seconds if necessary.

Jog in Place: Jog in position for 1 minute.
If low-impact activity suits you better, march for 1 minute with high knees in position.

Punching time: 1 minute
Punching is an excellent method to warm up the upper body and get the circulation flowing throughout the body.

Stand with your feet slightly wider than shoulder width apart and your knees slightly bent. Strengthen your core muscles to maintain your center steady. Punch out one arm at a time, keeping a consistent speed.

Knee Thrusters: Do 1 minute of knee thrusters. Begin by standing with your feet wider than shoulder-width apart and turning both feet in one way, allowing your hips to follow in a shallow lunge. The front knee is bent at 90 degrees, while the rear heel is elevated. Arms are held in front of the chest in a guard position.

Raise the back knee to hip height and bring the hands in toward the thigh. Repeat with the other foot on the floor.

Squat Basic: 1 Minute Squat
The basic squat will round up your warm-up. To maintain your hip flexors flexible, try to sink your glutes as low as possible.

Place your feet hip-distance apart and stand tall. All of your hips, knees, and toes should be pointed forward. Bend your knees and stretch your buttocks backwards, as if you were preparing to sit in a chair. Maintain your knees on your toes and your weight on your heels. Get back up.

The Elements of a Successful Workout

Workout Time: 15 Minutes
Do the exercises listed below for the prescribed amount of repetitions. Rest for 1 minute between exercises.

Squat Curl Knee Raise squat curl Biceps, glutes, and quads

Begin in a squat with your weight back on your heels and your arms extended next to your side, grasping dumbbells.

As you curl the weights to your shoulders, squeeze your glutes to press up and elevate your right knee.
Return to a squat stance by slowly lowering the weights. Rep with your left knee.
8 to 12 reps per side

Safety Recommendation

When you sit into each squat exercise, try to maintain your back straight and your chest open. While you curl, keep your elbows tight to your ribs.

Shoulders are the primary targets.
Begin with your feet hip-distance apart. Bring your elbows out to the side, arms in a goal post position, weights at the side of your head, and abs firm.
Slowly raise dumbbells until your arms are straight. Return to the starting position slowly and with control. Rep until you've completed the required amount of reps.

To work harder and develop balance, execute half the exercises on one foot, then switch to the other foot.

8 to 12 reps

Safety Recommendation

Directly above the shoulders, lift the weights. Allowing your arms to drift back may cause your back to arch. If you have trouble keeping excellent posture throughout this activity, do it while seated.

Triceps, back, and shoulders

Begin with your legs together and sit back into a small squat, working your abdominals. Arms are extended in front of the body, dumbbells at hip height, palms towards the ceiling.
Pull your elbows back beyond your hips, softly embracing your side body, until you feel your lats and triceps activate, then return forward with control.

8 to 12 reps Safety Tip

Maintain a neutral spine throughout this movement. Try not to arch your back or curve your spine. Maintain your attention on the floor a few feet in front of your toes.

Kneel on all fours on the floor (or an exercise mat if you have one). Extend one arm long behind you, draw in your abs, and stretch the opposing leg long behind you.
Rep on the opposite side.
8 to 10 reps per side

Safety Recommendation

Go slowly and steadily, briefly holding the arm and leg out before switching.

Glute Bridge Targets: Glutes and Hamstrings

Lay on your back with your knees bent and your feet flat and stacked beneath your knees.

As you elevate your hips to a bridge, engage your core and clench your glutes. Hold tightly and return to the mat with control.

To make it more difficult, perform this exercise with one leg at a time. While you thrust your hips up and down, lift the non-working leg into the air.

8 to 12 reps Safety Tip

To protect your neck, keep your gaze fixed on the ceiling.

Kneeling Shoulder Tap Push Up

Start in a kneeling plank position with hands on the ground below shoulders and back extended long to the knees.

Lower chest to the floor, keeping abs tight. As you push back up to the kneeling plank, tap your right hand on your left shoulder, then set it down.

Repeat the push-up, but as you rise, tap the left hand on the right shoulder. Keep abs tight throughout and don't allow the torso to tip to the side as you tap.

Reps: 8 to 12 push-ups total

Safety Tip

If your knees are uncomfortable, place a folded blanket under them for this move.

Start lying face down on the mat. Lift abs away from the mat to engage them and slide the shoulders down the back. The head is lifted in a low hover. Your body is one long line.

Using your back muscles and core, lift the chest away from the mat into extension as you exhale. Think of lengthening from the crown of the head.

Inhale and return back down to the mat slowly, getting longer through the spine as you go.

Reps: 8 to 12

Safety Tip

Skip this move if it causes pain in your back. If your back feels fine, you can add a challenge by performing the exercise with your arms out in front like superman.

Start lying on a mat with arms extended overhead, legs long, and feet flexed.
Inhale as you lift arms up and begin curling chin and chest forward. Exhale as you roll the entire torso up and over legs keeping abs engaged and reaching for toes.
Inhale as you begin rolling your spine back down one vertebra at a time and exhale as the upper portion of the back lower and arms reach the pack overhead. Repeat moving slowly and using the abdominals to lift and lower, not momentum.
Reps: 8 to 10

Safety Tip

If this is not comfortable on your back, bend the knees and do an abdominal crunch instead. With the feet flat on the floor, place your hands behind your head and curl the upper body off the floor. Lower back down and repeat.

Cool Down

Take five minutes to bring your heart rate down and your breathing back to normal. Walk in place or around the room or do some simple full-body stretches to relax and finish up your workout.

CHAPTER 5

How Chair Yoga can Help You

If you're looking for a gentle and accessible form of exercise that can improve your physical and mental wellbeing, consider incorporating Chair Yoga into your routine. Here's how this workout can help you:

Improve Flexibility and Range of Motion: Chair Yoga involves gentle stretches and movements that can help increase your flexibility and range of motion. By performing these exercises regularly, you can reduce stiffness and pain in your joints, which can be especially helpful if you have arthritis or other mobility issues.

Build Strength and Endurance: Even though Chair Yoga is a low-impact form of exercise, it can still help you build strength and endurance. Many of the poses involve engaging your core, back, and leg muscles, which can help improve your posture and balance.

Reduce Stress and Anxiety: Practicing Chair Yoga can also be a great way to reduce stress and anxiety. The deep breathing and relaxation techniques used in this workout can help calm your mind and body, reduce tension in your muscles, and promote feelings of inner peace and tranquility.

Improve Heart Health: Chair Yoga can also be beneficial for your cardiovascular system. Some of the poses involve gentle cardiovascular exercise, such as raising your arms overhead or doing seated twists, which can help improve your heart health and circulation.

Enhance Overall Wellbeing: Finally, incorporating Chair Yoga into your routine can have a positive impact on your overall wellbeing. By improving your physical health, reducing stress and anxiety, and promoting relaxation, this workout can help you feel more energized, focused, and confident in your daily life.

So if you're looking for a gentle yet effective form of exercise that can improve your physical and mental wellbeing, consider giving Chair Yoga a try. Whether you're new to fitness or looking to supplement your existing routine, this workout has something to offer everyone.

CHAPTER 6

Workout for Well-Being

Working out is a great way to promote physical, mental, and emotional well-being. Exercise not only helps to improve physical fitness and health, but it also has a positive impact on mental health and overall well-being.

Physical Benefits of Working Out

Regular exercise has numerous physical benefits that contribute to overall well-being. Exercise helps to improve cardiovascular health, strengthen muscles and bones, and improve balance and flexibility. Additionally, exercise helps to regulate weight and prevent chronic diseases such as diabetes, heart disease, and certain types of cancer.

Mental Benefits of Working Out

Working out also has a positive impact on mental health. Exercise is known to release endorphins, which are natural mood-boosters. Regular exercise has been shown to reduce stress and anxiety, improve sleep quality, and increase overall feelings of happiness and well-being. Exercise can also help to improve cognitive function and reduce the risk of developing dementia and other cognitive impairments.

Tips for Incorporating Exercise into Your Life

In order to reap the benefits of exercise for well-being, it is important to make it a regular part of your routine. Here are some tips for incorporating exercise into your life:

Find an activity you enjoy: The key to sticking with exercise is to find an activity that you enjoy. Whether it is running, cycling, swimming, or dancing, find an activity that makes you feel good and stick with it.

Make it a habit: Schedule exercise into your day just like any other important task. By making it a regular part of your routine, it will become a habit and you will be more likely to stick with it.

Start slow and gradually increase: If you are new to exercise, it is important to start slow and gradually increase the intensity and duration of your workouts. This will help to prevent injury and ensure that you enjoy the process.

Mix it up: It is important to mix up your workouts to prevent boredom and challenge your body. Try incorporating a variety of activities such as strength training, cardio, and flexibility exercises.

Set realistic goals: Setting realistic goals can help to keep you motivated and on track.

Whether it is running a 5K or completing a certain number of pushups, setting a goal can help to give you a sense of accomplishment and keep you focused.

Find a workout buddy: Exercising with a friend or family member can help to make it more fun and keep you accountable. Plus, it provides an opportunity for social interaction, which is also important for overall well-being.

General pain and recovery core workout for seniors

As we age, it is common for our bodies to experience aches and pains, particularly in our joints and muscles. These pains can make it difficult to stay active and maintain a healthy lifestyle. However, there are ways to alleviate these pains and improve mobility through chair yoga.

A core workout is an essential part of any exercise routine, and it is particularly important for seniors. Strong core muscles can improve balance, stability, and posture, which can prevent falls and reduce the risk of injury. Here are some general pain and recovery core exercises that can be done in a chair:

Seated Twist

Begin by sitting up straight in a chair with your feet flat on the floor. Place your left hand on your right knee and your right hand on the back of the chair. Inhale deeply and exhale as you twist your torso to the right. Hold the twist for a few seconds before returning to center. Repeat on the other side.

Leg Lifts

Sit up straight with your feet flat on the floor. Lift one leg up until it is parallel to the floor, then lower it back down. Repeat on the other leg. You can also try lifting both legs at the same time for an added challenge.

Knee Raises

Sit up straight with your feet flat on the floor. Lift one knee up towards your chest, then lower it back down. Repeat on the other leg. You can also try lifting both knees at the same time for an added challenge.

Seated Bicycle

Sit up straight with your feet flat on the floor. Lift one knee up towards your chest while simultaneously twisting your torso to bring the opposite elbow towards the knee. Repeat on the other side, alternating sides like you are pedaling a bicycle.

Seated Crunch

Sit up straight with your feet flat on the floor. Place your hands behind your head and slowly curl your torso forward, bringing your elbows towards your knees. Pause for a few seconds before slowly returning to the starting position.

Seated Side Bends

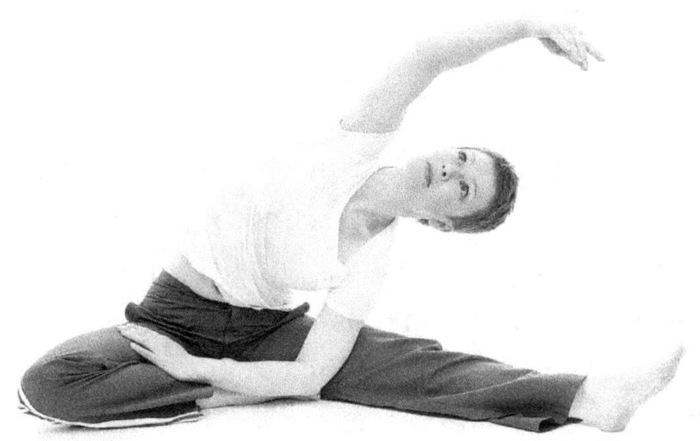

Sit up straight with your feet flat on the floor. Place your hands on your hips and lean to one side, bending at the waist. Hold the stretch for a few seconds before returning to center. Repeat on the other side.

Seated Plank

Sit up straight with your hands resting on the armrests of the chair. Lift your body up by pushing through your hands and straightening your arms. Hold the plank position for a few seconds before lowering your body back down.

These exercises are a great way to strengthen your core muscles and improve your overall fitness. They can also be done from the comfort of your own home using a chair as a prop. Remember to start slowly and gradually increase the difficulty of the exercises as your strength improves. Always listen to your body and stop if you feel any pain or discomfort. With regular practice, you will notice improvements in your mobility, balance, and overall well being.

Exercises to Perform If You Have Back Pain

Do you have a bad back? While breaking a sweat, these motions will help you recover and avoid additional damage.
Back discomfort may be excruciating. Many people experience chronic pain, ranging from tight shoulders caused by hunching over the computer to lower back aches caused by a herniated disc or a muscle strain.

A poor back may be both annoying and debilitating. Nonetheless, unless you're out of commission due to an acute accident, back pain should not interfere with your normal activities. Regular exercise, stretches, and strengthening can really help you heal from and avoid additional injuries. It's just a matter of determining which sorts of exercise are most suited to addressing ailments related to the spine.

HuffPost spoke with spine doctors and physical therapists on the best and safest back workouts. Here's what they say:

First, identify the problem.
The first step in treating back pain, according to Jaspal Singh, head of interventional spine at the department of rehabilitation medicine at Weill Cornell Medical, is determining the kind.

Singh suggested scheduling an appointment with a physiatrist, who can analyze your symptoms and ask you specific questions about your discomfort. Depending on the severity of the damage, some doctors may recommend imaging.

According to Singh, injuries to the discs between the bones of the spine are more prevalent in young individuals. If you suffer pain when you sneeze or cough, or when you bend forward or flex your spine, you may have a herniated disc.

If this is the case, you should avoid any activity that puts additional pressure on the disc, such as heavy lifting and high-impact exercises like running and leaping, as well as any motions that entail bending forward or leaning back, such as some forward folds in yoga, crunches, and situps. This can sometimes involve cycling, if your sitting position has your spine curved forward.

If it aches to sit but not to lean forward, you may have a muscle or joint strain rather than a disc problem. "The greatest method to decompress the spine when you're sitting is to remove the strain off it, so standing up, leaning back, or obtaining a sitting/standing workstation," Singh says.

Engage your upper back muscles gently.
If you have upper back or shoulder pain, Singh recommends resistance band rows, reverse snow angels, and scapular retraction – workouts that engage the mid-shoulder blades.

This will aid in the strengthening of the region and the prevention of future injuries. As Singh stated, begin with body weight or resistance bands before advancing to dumbbells or larger weights.

Swimming and other low-impact aerobic activities can help you heal from a back problem.
Swimming and other low-impact aerobic activities can help you heal from a back problem.
Choose low-impact cardio.
Low-impact cardio is good regardless of the sort of back pain you have.

Swimming, cycling (if seated with your spine straight, rather than leaning forward, which puts too much stress on the lower back), walking, and utilizing an elliptical machine are all advised by Singh. These are all excellent cardiovascular exercises that will keep your blood flowing and muscles supple without placing too much strain on your joints.

Running and leaping, as in calisthenics and other HIIT routines, can be too high-impact and strain the discs.

Work on your posture.
Try resistance bands and body-weight workouts, as well as yoga and pilates, if you want the core-and-glute-strengthening advantages of HIIT. So, first and foremost, you should improve your posture.

Many back problems are caused by bad posture, according to Lara Heimann, a physical therapist and founder of the LYT Yoga approach. These can cause "anterior pelvic tilt," in which the pelvis and hips shift forward, causing the spine to bend and producing muscle and joint imbalances.

"When people live with an anterior tilted pelvis routinely, it affects the back tissue, making the lower back shorter while the front lengthens, so the low back feels tight," Heimann explained. "It also positions your glutes in a position where the brain does not stimulate them to fire."

This causes weakening glutes and abdominal muscles, as well as additional tension on the lower back.

The good news is that there are methods for correcting alignment and building a strong, stable spine. Imagine your spine as a vertical line, like a plant, and your pelvic bowl as the plant's pot. Heimann stated that you want the bowl to be balanced, not tilted, so that the plant may grow strong and straight. "You're training your brain to move in a new way."

To achieve this alignment, try several positions and activities that engage your core, neutralize your pelvis, and stretch your spine.

Stand with your back to a wall, pressing your skull, shoulder blades, and sacrum (the area where the bottom of your spine meets the top of your buttocks) flat against the wall. You may also accomplish this by lying down with your skull, shoulder blades, and sacrum flat against the floor.

How to improve the strength of your core and glutes.

With a neutral pelvic posture, you may appropriately do activities that activate your core and glutes.

Heimann suggested wall squats and low bridges, in which you bend your knees in front of you and then elevate your hips, maintaining your pelvis neutral and your glutes tight. Be cautious not to pop your rib cage up, as this can throw your alignment off.

You may then try variants on the low bridge, such as a one-legged bridge with one leg straight and the other bent, and then swap. Heimann recommended holding each for a minute and doing it four times each day. You may also do a 30 count raise and lower.

Planks are an excellent approach to strengthen the core while maintaining the spine in neutral posture. Singh recommended against doing crunches or situps if you have back discomfort or an injury.

"Planks are a terrific method to maintain your core strength by working the most essential core muscle, the transverse abdominis," Singh added. They also activate the core "without exerting undue strain on the disc, joints, or muscles."

Place your forearms flat on a mat to do a perfect plank (or put your hands flat, directly under your shoulders). Maintain a straight back. Raise your head while maintaining your chin down and your neck in line with your back. Depending on your fitness level, hold for 30 seconds to a minute or two minutes. Once you've mastered the plank, you may experiment with different variants.

Singh also suggests Supermans, lotsus yoga poses, and cat-cow yoga poses.

And a good rule of thumb, according to Singh, is to listen to your body. If something doesn't feel right, especially if it's producing severe, shooting pain, it's time to stop.

Nevertheless, if you focus on correcting your alignment, strengthening your core, and maintaining a low-impact exercise routine, you will be on the road to greater spine health.

"These are useful maneuvers that may be transferred into daily life and other athletics," Heimann explained. "You're training the brain to move differently and preparing the body to do new things safely."

Losing weight is a common goal for many people, and there are many ways to approach it. One of the most effective methods is through exercise. A weight loss workout is a great way to burn calories, increase metabolism, and improve overall health. In this chapter, we will discuss the benefits of exercise for weight loss and provide a comprehensive guide to creating an effective weight loss workout.

Benefits of Exercise for Weight Loss:

There are several benefits of exercise for weight loss, including:

Increased Calorie Burn: Exercise helps you burn calories, which is essential for weight loss. When you engage in physical activity, your body burns calories to fuel the movement. The more intense the exercise, the more calories you burn.

Increased Metabolism: Exercise also helps to increase your metabolism. A faster metabolism means your body burns calories more efficiently, even when you're at rest. This can help you lose weight faster and more effectively.

Improved Cardiovascular Health: Exercise is also good for your heart and cardiovascular health. Regular exercise can help to reduce the risk of heart disease and other health problems.

Reduced Stress: Exercise can also help to reduce stress, which is a common trigger for overeating and weight gain.

Creating a Weight Loss Workout:

When creating a weight loss workout, there are several factors to consider. These include:

Cardiovascular Exercise: Cardiovascular exercise is essential for weight loss. It burns calories and helps to increase your metabolism.

Examples of cardio exercise include running, cycling, swimming, and jumping rope.

Strength Training: Strength training is also important for weight loss. It helps to build muscle, which in turn increases your metabolism. Examples of strength training exercises include weightlifting, push-ups, and squats.

High-Intensity Interval Training: High-Intensity Interval Training (HIIT) is a form of cardio exercise that involves short bursts of intense activity followed by periods of rest. It is an effective way to burn calories and increase your metabolism.

Flexibility Training: Flexibility training, such as yoga or Pilates, can help to improve your range of motion and reduce the risk of injury.

Sample Weight Loss Workout:

- Here is a sample weight loss workout that incorporates cardiovascular exercise, strength training, and HIIT:

- Warm-up: 5-10 minutes of light cardio, such as jogging or jumping jacks.

- Cardiovascular Exercise: 20-30 minutes of moderate to high-intensity cardio, such as running, cycling, or swimming

- Strength Training: 20-30 minutes of strength training, such as weightlifting or bodyweight exercises.
  -

- HIIT: 10-15 minutes of HIIT, such as sprinting or jumping rope.
  -

- Cool-down: 5-10 minutes of light cardio, such as walking or stretching.

Tips for Success:

*Here are some tips to help you succeed with your
weight loss workout:*

Set Realistic Goals: Set realistic goals for
your weight loss workout. Don't expect to lose a
significant amount of weight in a short period of
time. Aim for a gradual, sustainable weight loss
of 1-2 pounds per week.

Stay Consistent: Consistency is key when it
comes to weight loss. Try to exercise at least
three to four times per week.

Mix It Up: Don't do the same workout every
day. Mix it up to keep things interesting and
challenging.

Fuel Your Body: Make sure to fuel your body
with healthy foods to support your weight loss
goals.

A weight loss workout can be a highly effective way to lose weight and improve your overall health. By incorporating cardiovascular exercise, strength training, and HIIT into your routine, you can burn calories, increase your metabolism, and achieve your goals.

Workout for Knee Injury

Knee injuries are common among athletes and people who engage in physical activity. Knee injuries can be caused by a variety of factors, including overuse, traumatic injury, and degenerative conditions. One of the most effective ways to recover from a knee injury is through exercise. In this chapter, we will discuss the benefits of exercise for knee injury recovery and provide a comprehensive guide to creating an effective workout for knee injury.

Benefits of Exercise for Knee Injury Recovery:

There are several benefits of exercise for knee injury recovery, including:

Improved Range of Motion: Exercise can help to improve range of motion in the knee joint. This can help to reduce pain and stiffness and improve overall function.

Increased Strength: Exercise can help to increase strength in the muscles surrounding the knee joint. Stronger muscles can help to support the joint and reduce the risk of further injury.

Reduced Pain: Exercise can help to reduce pain associated with knee injuries. This is because exercise releases endorphins, which are natural painkillers.

Improved Balance and Stability: Exercise can help to improve balance and stability, which can reduce the risk of falls and further injury.

Creating a Workout for Knee Injury:

When creating a workout for knee injury, there are several factors to consider. These include:

Low-Impact Exercises: Low-impact exercises are ideal for knee injury recovery. These exercises are gentle on the knee joint and can help to improve range of motion and strength without causing further injury. Examples of low-impact exercises include walking, cycling, swimming, and yoga.

Strengthening Exercises: Strengthening exercises are also important for knee injury recovery. These exercises help to build strength in the muscles surrounding the knee joint, which can help to support the joint and reduce the risk of further injury. Examples of strengthening exercises include leg presses, hamstring curls, and calf raises.

Stretching Exercises: Stretching exercises can help to improve range of motion in the knee joint and reduce stiffness and pain. Examples of stretching exercises include quad stretches, hamstring stretches, and calf stretches.

Balance and Stability Exercises: Balance and stability exercises can help to improve balance and reduce the risk of falls and further injury. Examples of balance and stability exercises include standing on one leg, heel-to-toe walking, and using a balance board.

Sample Workout for Knee Injury:

Here is a sample workout for knee injury that incorporates low-impact exercises, strengthening exercises, stretching exercises, and balance and stability exercises:

- Warm-up: 5-10 minutes of light cardio, such as walking or cycling.

- Low-Impact Exercise: 20-30 minutes of low-impact exercise, such as walking, cycling, or swimming.

- Strengthening Exercise: 20-30 minutes of strengthening exercise, such as leg presses, hamstring curls, and calf raises.

- Stretching Exercise: 10-15 minutes of stretching exercise, such as quad stretches, hamstring stretches, and calf stretches.

- Balance and Stability Exercise: 10-15 minutes of balance and stability exercise, such as standing on one leg, heel-to-toe walking, and using a balance board.

- Cool-down: 5-10 minutes of light cardio, such as walking or stretching.

Tips for Success:

Here are some tips to help you succeed with your knee injury workout:

Consult with Your Doctor: Before starting any exercise program for knee injury, consult with your doctor or physical therapist to ensure that the program is safe and appropriate for your specific injury.

Start Slowly: If you are new to exercise or have not exercised in a while, start slowly and gradually increase the intensity and duration of your workouts.

Listen to Your Body: If you experience pain or discomfort during exercise.

Wheelchair workout

Physical activity is essential for maintaining overall health and wellness, regardless of physical ability. For individuals who use wheelchairs, finding appropriate workout options can be challenging. However, there are numerous exercises and workout options that can be tailored to an individual's specific abilities and limitations. In this chapter, we will discuss the benefits of exercise for wheelchair users and provide a comprehensive guide to creating an effective wheelchair workout.

Benefits of Exercise for Wheelchair Users:

Physical activity offers numerous benefits for individuals who use wheelchairs, including:

Improved Cardiovascular Health: Exercise can help to improve cardiovascular health, which is important for individuals who use wheelchairs since they may have limited mobility.

Increased Strength and Endurance: Exercise can help to increase strength and endurance, which can improve overall function and make everyday tasks easier.

Reduced Risk of Secondary Conditions: Exercise can help to reduce the risk of secondary conditions associated with wheelchair use, such as pressure sores, muscle atrophy, and osteoporosis.

Improved Mental Health: Exercise can help to improve mental health by reducing stress, anxiety, and depression.

Creating a Workout for Wheelchair Users:

When creating a workout for wheelchair users, there are several factors to consider. These include:

Range of Motion Exercises: Range of motion exercises are important for maintaining flexibility and preventing muscle contractures.

Examples of range of motion exercises for wheelchair users include arm circles, shoulder rolls, and wrist stretches.

Strengthening Exercises: Strengthening exercises can help to increase strength and improve overall function. Examples of strengthening exercises for wheelchair users include resistance band exercises, seated dumbbell exercises, and push-ups from the wheelchair.

Cardiovascular Exercises: Cardiovascular exercises are important for improving heart health and increasing endurance. Examples of cardiovascular exercises for wheelchair users include hand cycling, wheelchair basketball, and wheelchair racing.

Balance and Coordination Exercises: Balance and coordination exercises can help to improve stability and reduce the risk of falls. Examples of balance and coordination exercises for wheelchair users include weight shifting, reaching exercises, and trunk rotations.

Sample Workout for Wheelchair Users:

Here is a sample workout for wheelchair users that incorporates range of motion exercises, strengthening exercises, cardiovascular exercises, and balance and coordination exercises:

- Warm-up: 5-10 minutes of light cardio, such as hand cycling or wheelchair basketball.

- Range of Motion Exercise: 10-15 minutes of range of motion exercises, such as arm circles, shoulder rolls, and wrist stretches.

- Strengthening Exercise: 20-30 minutes of strengthening exercise, such as resistance band exercises, seated dumbbell exercises, and push-ups from the wheelchair.

- Cardiovascular Exercise: 20-30 minutes of cardiovascular exercise, such as hand cycling, wheelchair basketball, or wheelchair racing.

- Balance and Coordination Exercise: 10-15 minutes of balance and coordination exercises, such as weight shifting, reaching exercises, and trunk rotations.

- Cool-down: 5-10 minutes of light cardio, such as hand cycling or wheelchair basketball.

Tips for Success:

Here are some tips to help you succeed with your wheelchair workout:

Consult with Your Doctor: Before starting any exercise program, consult with your doctor or physical therapist to ensure that the program is safe and appropriate for your specific needs.

Start Slowly: If you are new to exercise or have not exercised in a while, start slowly and gradually increase the intensity and duration of your workouts.

Use Proper Technique: Using proper technique is essential for preventing injury and ensuring that you get the most out of your workouts. Work with a certified personal trainer or physical therapist to learn proper technique.

Listen to Your Body: If you experience pain or discomfort during exercise, stop and rest.

Working out is an important aspect of promoting overall well-being. It has numerous physical, mental, and emotional benefits that can improve quality of life. By incorporating exercise into your routine and making it a regular habit, you can reap the benefits of exercise and enjoy a healthier, happier life.

CHAPTER 7

Physical, Mental and Emotional Benefits of Chair Yoga

Yoga is a physical, mental, and spiritual practice that originated in ancient India thousands of years ago. It has become increasingly popular in Western cultures as a way to improve physical fitness, reduce stress, and promote overall wellness. One form of yoga that has gained popularity in recent years is chair yoga, which is a modified form of traditional yoga that is performed while sitting on a chair. In this chapter, we will explore the physical, mental, and emotional benefits of chair yoga.

Physical Benefits of Chair Yoga

Chair yoga offers many physical benefits, including improved flexibility, strength, and balance. Since chair yoga is performed while seated, it is an ideal form of exercise for those who have limited mobility, injuries, or other health conditions that make it difficult to perform traditional yoga poses.

Improved Flexibility: Chair yoga can help improve flexibility by stretching and lengthening muscles. The practice of chair yoga poses such as seated twists, forward folds, and side stretches can help to improve the range of motion in the spine, hips, shoulders, and neck.

Increased Strength: Chair yoga also helps to increase muscle strength. Many of the poses involve holding the body in a specific position, which can help to build strength in the core, arms, and legs. Additionally, using resistance bands or weights during chair yoga can further enhance strength building.

Improved Balance: Chair yoga can also help to improve balance, which is essential for maintaining stability and preventing falls. Many chair yoga poses involve sitting on one leg or standing on one leg while holding onto the chair for support. These poses can help to strengthen the muscles that are responsible for balance and improve proprioception, which is the body's ability to sense its position in space.

Mental Benefits of Chair Yoga

In addition to its physical benefits, chair yoga can also have a positive impact on mental health. Regular practice of chair yoga can help to reduce stress, improve focus, and promote feelings of calm and relaxation.

Stress Reduction: Chair yoga is a form of mindfulness practice that involves focusing on the breath and being present in the moment. This can help to reduce stress and anxiety by calming the mind and promoting a sense of relaxation.

Improved Focus: Chair yoga also helps to improve focus and concentration by bringing attention to the body and breath. This can help to reduce distractions and improve mental clarity.

Increased Relaxation: Chair yoga can also help to promote feelings of calm and relaxation by activating the parasympathetic nervous system, which is responsible for the body's "rest and digest" response. This can help to lower heart rate and blood pressure, reduce muscle tension, and promote overall feelings of well-being.

Emotional Benefits of Chair Yoga

Chair yoga can also have a positive impact on emotional health by promoting self-awareness, self-esteem, and a sense of connection with others.

Self-Awareness: Chair yoga involves bringing attention to the body and breath, which can help to improve self-awareness and promote a sense of mindfulness. This can help to increase self-esteem and confidence by improving the ability to recognize and regulate emotions.

Self-Esteem: Chair yoga can also help to promote self-esteem by providing a sense of accomplishment and empowerment. By practicing and mastering new poses, individuals can feel a sense of pride and confidence in their abilities.

Connection with Others: Chair yoga can also help to promote a sense of connection with others by providing a supportive and inclusive environment. Practicing yoga with others can help to reduce feelings of isolation and promote social connection.

Chair yoga is a modified form of traditional yoga that can provide many physical, mental, and emotional benefits. Whether you are an older adult, have limited mobility, or are simply looking for a more gentle form of exercise, chair yoga is for you.

Conclusion

"Ageless Yoga" is a valuable resource for seniors looking to improve their physical and mental well-being. This book provides a comprehensive guide to chair yoga, a form of yoga that is accessible to seniors of all abilities and fitness levels. The author, a certified yoga instructor, has designed each yoga sequence to provide a safe and effective workout that is tailored to the needs of seniors.

One of the strengths of this book is its focus on the benefits of chair yoga for seniors. The author does an excellent job of explaining how chair yoga can improve flexibility, balance, strength, and mental health. For seniors who may be hesitant to try yoga, this book provides a compelling case for why chair yoga is an ideal form of exercise for them.

Another strength of this book is its accessibility. The author uses clear and concise language to explain each yoga pose, and the accompanying photographs make it easy to understand how to perform each pose correctly. The author also provides modifications for each pose, making it possible for seniors with limited mobility to participate in the yoga sequences.

In addition to the physical benefits of chair yoga, the author also emphasizes the mental health benefits of this form of exercise. Chair yoga can be a powerful tool for reducing stress and anxiety, improving sleep quality, and enhancing overall well-being. By incorporating mindfulness and relaxation techniques into each yoga sequence, the author helps seniors to cultivate a sense of calm and inner peace.

Throughout the book, the author emphasizes the importance of safety when practicing chair yoga. Seniors may have unique physical limitations or health concerns that require modifications to their yoga practice. The author provides clear guidance on how to adapt each pose to meet the needs of seniors, and encourages readers to listen to their bodies and make adjustments as necessary.

One of the unique features of this book is the inclusion of specific yoga sequences for common health concerns that seniors may experience. For example, the author provides sequences for improving balance, relieving joint pain, and reducing anxiety. By tailoring the yoga sequences to address specific health concerns, the author makes it easy for seniors to incorporate chair yoga into their daily routine as a form of self-care.

Overall, "Chair Yoga for Seniors" is an excellent resource for seniors looking to improve their physical and mental well-being. The author provides a clear and comprehensive guide to chair yoga, emphasizing the benefits of this form of exercise for seniors. The book is accessible and easy to understand, with modifications provided for each pose to ensure that seniors of all abilities can participate. By incorporating mindfulness and relaxation techniques into each yoga sequence, the author helps seniors to cultivate a sense of calm and inner peace, which can be a powerful tool for improving overall well-being.

One potential limitation of this book is that it is focused specifically on chair yoga. While chair yoga is an ideal form of exercise for many seniors, some may be interested in exploring other forms of yoga as well. However, for seniors who are specifically looking for a low-impact form of exercise that can be done from the comfort of their own home, chair yoga is an excellent choice.

In conclusion, "Chair Yoga for Seniors" is a valuable resource for seniors looking to improve their physical and mental well-being. The author provides a comprehensive guide to chair yoga, emphasizing the benefits of this form of exercise for seniors. The book is accessible and easy to understand, with modifications provided for each pose to ensure that seniors of all abilities can participate. By incorporating mindfulness and relaxation techniques into each yoga sequence, the author helps seniors to cultivate a sense of calm and inner peace, which can be a powerful tool for improving overall well-being. This book is a must-read for seniors who are looking for an effective and accessible form of exercise that can help them to maintain their physical and mental health as they age.